Air Pollution and Health

AIR POLLUTION REVIEWS

Series Editor: Robert L. Maynard
(Department of Health, Skipton House, London, U.K.)

Air Pollution Reviews — Vol. 3

Air Pollution and Health

Jon Ayres
University of Aberdeen, UK

Robert Maynard
UK Department of Health, UK

Roy Richards
University of Cardiff, UK

Imperial College Press

ICP

Published by

Imperial College Press
57 Shelton Street
Covent Garden
London WC2H 9HE

Distributed by

World Scientific Publishing Co. Pte. Ltd.
5 Toh Tuck Link, Singapore 596224
USA office: 27 Warren Street, Suite 401-402, Hackensack, NJ 07601
UK office: 57 Shelton Street, Covent Garden, London WC2H 9HE

British Library Cataloguing-in-Publication Data
A catalogue record for this book is available from the British Library.

The image on the front cover courtesy of Peter M. Ayres

AIR POLLUTION AND HEALTH
Air Pollution Reviews — Vol. 3

ISBN   1-86094-191-5

Printed in Singapore by B & JO Enterprise

CONTRIBUTORS

Jon G Ayres
Environmental & Occupational
Medicine
Liberty Safe Work Research
Centre
University of Aberdeen
Foresterhill Road
Aberdeen AB25 2ZP

Dominique Balharry
School of Biosciences
Cardiff University
Museum Avenue
Cardiff CF10 3US
Wales

Kelly A Bérubé PhD FRMS
Cardiff School of Biosciences
Biomedical Building
Museum Avenue
PO Box 911
Cardiff CF10 3US

Lung Chi Chen
Department of Environmental
Medicine
New York University School
of Medicine
57 old Forge Road
Tuxedo
NY 10987
USA

Ken Donaldson
MRC/University of Edinburgh
Centre for Inflammation
Research
The Queen's Medical
Research Institute
47 Little France Crescent
Edinburgh, EH16 4TJ

Ron Eccles
Director
Common Cold Centre
Cardiff School of Biosciences
Biomedical Building
Museum Avenue
Cardiff CF10 3US, UK

Paul Elliott
Imperial College School
of Medicine
Department of Epidemiology
& Public Health
St. Mary's Campus
Norfolk Place
London W2 1PG

Steven Faux
MRC Toxicology Unit
Hodgkin Building
University of Leicester
Leicester LE1 9HN

Patrick Hayden
MatTek Corporation
200 Homer Avenue
Ashland
Massachusetts
01721 USA

Martina Hicks
School of Biosciences
Cardiff University
Museum Avenue
Cardiff CF10 3US
Wales

A E M De Hollander
Dept of Chronic Disease &
Environmental Epidemiology
National Institute of Public
Health & the Environment
PO Box 1
3720 B A Bilthoven
The Netherlands

Timothy Jones
School of Earth, Ocean and
Planetary Sciences
Cardiff University
Park Place
Cardiff CF10 3YE, Wales

Johan M Melse
Dept of Chronic Disease &
Environmental Epidemiology
National Institute of Public
Health & the Environment
PO Box 1
3720 B A Bilthoven
The Netherlands

Luciano Merolla
School of Biosciences
Cardiff University
Museum Avenue
Cardiff CF10 3US
Wales

Teresa Moreno
Instituto de Ciencieas de la
Tierra "Jaume Almera"
Consejo Superior de
Investigaciones Cientificas
C/Lluis Sole I Sabaris s/n
08028 Barcelona
Spain

William NcNee
Centre for Inflammation
Research
University of Edinburgh
The Queen's Medical
Research Institute
47 Little France Crescent
Edinburgh, EH16 4TJ

Helen C. Routledge
Specialist Registrar
Department of Cardiology
Birmingham Heartlands
NHS Trust
Birmingham B9 5ST

Richard B. Schlesinger
Department of Biological
Sciences and Environmental
Science Program
Pace University
1 Pace Plaza
New York, NY 10038
USA

Keith Sexton
School of Biosciences
Cardiff University
Museum Avenue
Cardiff CF10 3US
Wales

Vicki Stone
Biomedicine Research Group
Napier University
10 Colinton Road
Edinburgh

Cynthia Timblin
Arti Shukla
Brooke Mossman
Department of Pathology
University of Vermont
Burlington
Vermont 05045 USA

PREFACE

The literature on air pollution and its effect on health has burgeoned over the last 15 to 20 years, triggered by the development of time-series methods and the seminal Six Cities Study in the United States, which prompted realisation that despite Clean Air Acts aimed at controlling industrial and domestic emissions, pollution was having an impact on health. Since then, the field has expanded and the increasing complexity of the issues raised has become apparent. Today, many robust criticisms of the science to date have been greeted with equally robust rebuttals and modifications of methodology, but the message remains the same. Air pollution affects populations throughout the world, having a significant impact on public health. An important source of these pollutants is the motor vehicle.

In our attempt to address some of the issues within the field in this volume, it is clear that there is sufficient material to fill many volumes. In this context, we decided to address a number of issues which have either been neglected or which pose important critical questions.

We begin with the role of the nose of modulating or initiating responses to air pollutants, move through the epidemiological and experimental evidence that cardiac function is disturbed by pollution, and then address the question of point sources as opposed to area sources when trying to apportion exposure sources with respect to specific health effects. New work on the structure of particles and their toxicology then leads to a chapter addressing how best we might determine particle toxicity in the future. This is of particular relevance at present in view of the increasing concerns regarding manufactured nano-materials. The volume concludes with a new approach to an assessment of the health impacts of air pollution — an area where policy developers keenly feel the need, when determining how best to address air pollution control. We hope that you will find some of these areas useful.

We are very grateful to the patience and tolerance of authors in putting together this volume. We take complete responsibility of any typographical errors that there may be within the text.

Prof. Jon G Ayres
University of Aberdeen

and

Dr. Robert Maynard
UK Department of Health

CONTENTS

*Kelly Bérubé, Dominique Balharry, Timothy Jones,
Teresa Moreno, Patrick Hayden, Keith Sexton,
Martina Hicks, Luciano Merolla, Cynthia Timblin,
Arti Shukla and Brooke Mossman*

CHAPTER 1

THE ROLE OF THE NOSE IN HEALTH AND DISEASE

Ron Eccles

1. Introduction

The nose is strategically situated at the entrance of the airway and acts as an air conditioner to condition the inspired air, before it reaches the more delicate gas exchange areas of the lungs. The average adult inhales around 10–20,000 litres of air (about 15 kilos of air) each day, which in mass is much more than the daily intake of food and water. The nose acts as an effective filter and gas scrubber and much of the suspended particulate matter and soluble gases in the inspired air are deposited in the nose (Witek, 1993). The air conditioning function of the nose exposes the nasal epithelium to a continuous threat of irritation, damage and infection, as the inspired air often contains pollutants such as ozone and sulphur dioxide, and pathogenic organisms such as viruses, bacteria, fungi and yeasts. The nasal epithelium has a great capacity to withstand the damaging effects of inspired air and the nasal defences and immune response resist and overcome infection. In this chapter, I will discuss how the nose protects the lower airways from the damaging effects of the inspired air, by describing the physiological mechanisms which defend the airway. I will also describe in general terms the effects of pollutants on the nose to illustrate how air pollution can cause nasal symptoms and nasal disease.

2. The Nose as a Defender of the Airway

The nose defends the airway in several ways; by acting as an air conditioner to warm, filter and humidify the inspired air so that clean air which is fully saturated with water vapour at a temperature of 37°C is delivered to the lungs; by clearing deposited particulate matter and dissolved gases in mucus which is swallowed and then removed by the digestive system; by detecting potentially noxious substances and initiating respiratory reflexes to clear the nose and prevent inspiration of the substances into the lungs; by absorbing and neutralising soluble gases which could harm the lungs; by neutralising infectious organisms and preventing infection of the lower airways. These defence mechanisms are illustrated in Fig. 1 and will be discussed in detail below.

2.1. *Filtration of Suspended Particulate Matter*

The nose acts as a very efficient filter of suspended particulate matter and most suspended matter is either deposited in the nose or

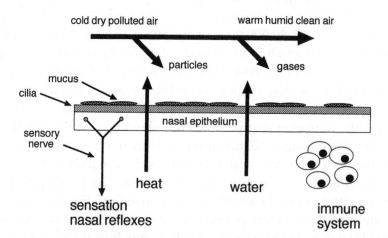

Fig. 1. Air conditioning and nasal defence mechanisms. Cold dry polluted air is conditioned to warm humid clean air by the nose. Particulate matter is deposited on the moving blanket of mucus and soluble gases are absorbed in the fluid layer lining the nose. Sensory nerves monitor the composition of the inspired air and trigger protective reflexes. Circulating leukocytes initiate specific and non specific immune responses to viruses and bacteria which penetrate the nasal epithelium.

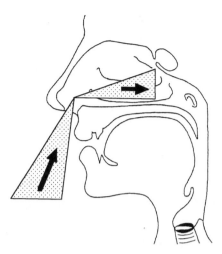

Fig. 2. Filtration of suspended particulate matter occurs at the anterior part of the nose where the airflow changes direction by 90 and decelerates as the air stream leaves the narrow nasal valve area to enter the nasal cavity. The shaded area represents the nasal air stream as it is funnelled through the nasal valve area.

breathed in and out without respiratory deposition. The filtration mechanism of the nose is firstly related to a sudden change in the direction of nasal airflow, as the air stream passes upwards through the nasal vestibule and then turns through 90° to enter the nasal cavity as shown in Fig. 2. The sudden change in the direction of nasal airflow tends to spin suspended matter out of the main air stream and onto the surface of the nasal epithelium. Secondly, there is an acceleration of the airflow as it passes through the nasal valve region, which is the narrowest part of the nose, and then a deceleration of airflow as the air stream enters the nasal cavity. The changes in direction and velocity of the air stream occur over the same area of the nose, at the level of the anterior end of the inferior turbinate and the slowing of the airflow at this point deposits particulate matter onto the nasal epithelium.

Much of the work of breathing is related to nasal filtration, as the nasal valve area forms the narrowest cross-sectional area of the whole airway at around $30\,\mathrm{mm}^2$ (Cole, 1982a), and this presents a considerable resistance to nasal airflow. Nasal airway resistance contributes up to two thirds of the total airway resistance and the work costs required from the respiratory muscles to move the airflow through the nasal valve area is the price that is paid for the filtration of the inspired air.

At very low levels of airflow, nasal airflow may be laminar, but for the greater part of the respiratory cycle, the airflow is turbulent with greater turbulence during inspiration than expiration (Wheatley et al., 1991). The twisting course of nasal airflow with changes in both velocity and direction ensure that nasal airflow is mainly turbulent, and this is important for proper conditioning and mixing of the inspired air. If the nasal airflow was mainly laminar, then only the portion of air directly in contact with the nasal epithelium would be conditioned by the exchange of heat and water.

The tendency for a particle suspended in the air stream to be deposited in the nose is determined by factors such as its physical size, shape, density and hygroscopicity. The physical size, shape and density of a particle can be quantified as the aerodynamic equivalent diameter of a particle (AED). Thus, regardless of size, shape or density, its AED refers to its behaviour in the air stream, if it were of unit density, spherical and of the stated diameter. Thus, a particle having an AED of 5 um may be smaller than this, but of a higher density or of a shape other than spherical. Particles with an AED larger than 180 um are virtually non-inspirable, whereas a proportion of particles with an AED smaller than that will be inspired. At an AED of ~ 30, 10 and 2.5 um, about 50, 70 and 90% of the particles will be inspired. During nose breathing, the majority of particles larger than 15 um AED are deposited in the upper respiratory tract, but with mouth breathing, some of these will penetrate into the trachea. Particles above 2.5 um AED are primarily deposited in the trachea and bronchi, whereas those below 2.5 um AED predominantly penetrate into the gas exchange region of the lungs (Andersen and Molhave, 1982).

2.2. Humidification of Inspired Air

The humidity of the air around us affects the evaporation of water from the skin and respiratory tract, and this is important for thermoregulation as the loss of heat from the body surface is limited when air humidity is high. Despite the fact that the upper airways condition the inspired air by increasing its humidity so that air reaching the lungs is saturated with water, we often feel uncomfortable when the humidity of the air around us is high. This may be partly related to feeling "hot and sticky", but it may also be related to the fact that we often have a sensation of "nasal stuffiness" when breathing air of high humidity, as the inspiratory nasal airflow does not provide the same cooling sensation of breathing.

The humidity of inhaled air may vary from 0.000002% to 4.5% by volume, with the lowest values measured at high altitudes or over the antarctic plateau and the highest values in the equatorial regions near shallow bodies of water (Andersen and Molhave, 1982).

The capacity of the upper airways to humidify the inspired air is very great and no drying of the nasal mucous membrane is seen after prolonged exposure to dry air. The inhaled air rapidly reaches saturation with water vapour, as it passes through the nose and upper airways so that by the level of the trachea, it is completely saturated. This saturation of the inhaled air is achieved despite a wide range of ambient air temperatures and humidity (Cole, 1982b). The water required for the humidification of the inhaled air is provided mainly by nasal glandular secretions, although it is unknown if there are any control mechanisms linking the water requirement for air conditioning and the rate of glandular secretion. It is possible that changes in the osmolarity of the thin layer of the nasal fluid control the movement of water across the nasal epithelium and that there is balance between water loss and the replenishment of water in the nasal fluid.

The humidification of the inspired air may also influence the filtration of particulate matter from the inspired air, since the hydration of hygroscopic particulate matter may cause the particles to swell and increase their AED. Water is lost from the surface of the nasal epithelium during inspiration, as it contributes to the humidification of the inspired air and the nasal epithelium is cooled, as it gives up heat both for warming the inspired air and by being associated with evaporation of water. During expiration, warm and fully saturated air passes through the cooler nasal airway and some water may be reclaimed from the expired air by condensation onto the cooler nasal epithelium. In cold weather, this condensed water may drip from the nose.

2.3. The Nose as a Heat Exchanger

The nasal epithelium has a complex network of blood vessels with a relatively high blood flow and the nose acts as a heat exchanger, so that over a wide range of ambient temperatures, the temperature of the inspired air is brought close to body temperature by the time it leaves the nose. In extremely cold climates, there may be further warming of the inspired air along the trachea, so that by the time the air reaches the lungs, the temperature is close to 37°C (Cole, 1982b). In temperate laboratory conditions, the temperature of the nasal epithelium is around 30°C immediately after inspiration and rises to 32°C immediately after expiration and the temperature of the expired air is close to 32°C.

2.4. Mucociliary Clearance

The thin layer of mucus and water covering the nasal epithelium is of vital importance for nasal defence against infection and the damaging effects of air pollution. The blanket of water and mucus overlying the nasal epithelium can be thought of as a conveyor belt continuously trapping and transporting particulate matter and dissolved gases from the nose to the nasopharynx where the mucus is swallowed.

In health, the ciliated epithelium of the nasal epithelium is covered with a thin layer of fluid and mucus. The cilia beat in a watery periciliary fluid, and overlying this is a layer of thick viscous mucus. It is the mucus rather than the periciliary fluid which is propelled at a rate of 3–25 mm/min, by the action of the cilia which beat at a rate of 1000 times per minute (Proctor, 1982). The mucus does not form a continuous sheet overlying the ciliated epithelium, but consists of irregular patches which sweep the epithelium clean as they propell along the surface.

Although we often refer to the nasal fluid as nasal secretions, only the component derived from nasal glands and goblet cells is actually "secreted" in the sense that it is derived from glandular cells. Nasal airway lining fluid is a mixture of elements derived from four sources (Eccles, 1983).

(1) Seromucous glands within the nasal epithelium.
(2) Goblet cells distributed along the surface of the nasal epithelium.

(3) Plasma exudate from capillaries and veins within the nasal epithelium.
(4) Cell debris from leukocytes and epithelial cells.

To these sources of airway lining fluid, one could also add contributions from the Bowman's glands of the olfactory epithelium and from the lacrimal glands via the nasolacrimal duct.

The seromucous glands are found deep within the nasal epithelium and the secretions flow onto the surface of the epithelium via large ducts. These glands are innervated by cholinergic parasympathetic nerve fibres and nasal irritation causes a profuse watery reflex nasal secretion via a trigeminal nerve reflex. Nasal irritation associated with inspired dust or at the start of a common cold infection triggers sneezing and a watery nasal secretion acts as defensive measures which help to expel and wash out the source of irritation.

Goblet cells are distributed throughout the surface of the respiratory epithelium and they contain mucus granules composed of high molecular weight mucus glycoproteins (mucins). Mucins are tightly packed in the intracellular granules and the release of mucins may be via a combination of merocrine and apocrine secretion (Rogers, 1994). Discharge of mucus occurs in a matter of tens of milliseconds and the granules increase in size many hundredfold, as they contact the airway lining fluid. Mucus discharge occurs in response to a wide variety of stimuli such as irritant gases, inflammatory mediators and infection, and there is some evidence that secretion is under the control of sensory nerve endings via neuropeptide release (Kuo *et al.*, 1990).

The nasal capillaries and venous sinuses contain small pores or fenestrae on the side facing the nasal epithelium, and these pores are believed to be the source of a nasal plasma exudate (Grevers, 1993). It has been proposed that exudation of plasma is a first line of respiratory defence (Persson *et al.*, 1991). In rhinitis, a major component of the nasal fluid may be due to an outpouring of plasma from the nasal blood vessels.

Nasal mucociliary clearance can be measured in man by placing a particle of saccharin on the anterior end of the inferior turbinate and timing the onset of a sweet taste when the saccharin reaches the pharynx and is swallowed. The rate of mucociliary clearance as measured by saccharin transport or other methods has a wide normal range, and is quoted as between 1–20 mm/min, with an average rat of 6 mm/min (Proctor, 1982) or as a clearance time of 7–11 min (Moriaty *et al.*, 1991). It is not clear why there should be such a large range for mucociliary clearance in normal healthy subjects, but this may be related to a previous history of upper respiratory tract infection, which is not always well documented in studies on mucociliary clearance.

The airway lining fluid of the nose has an important role in respiratory defence. The bacteriostatic proteins lactoferrin and lysozyme inhibit the growth of bacteria in the nose, and secretory antibodies help to prevent and limit viral infections. More recently, it has been shown that nasal airway lining fluid contains antioxidants such as uric acid and glutathione, which limit oxidative damage from air pollutants such as ozone (Cross *et al.*, 1994; Housley *et al.*, 1995).

2.5. *Innervation of the Nose and Nasal Reflexes*

The nose is ideally situated at the entrance to the respiratory tract to sample the inspired airstream and to detect chemical and physical irritants which could damage the airway. The sensory innervation of the nose is mainly supplied by the olfactory and trigeminal nerves (Eccles, 1982). The olfactory nerves enter the nose through the cribriform plate and form a distinct olfactory area. Most of the sensory nerves to the nasal epithelium and nasal vestibule are supplied by two branches of the trigeminal nerve, i.e. the ophthalmic and maxillary nerves.

The olfactory area acts as a long-distance chemoreceptor, sampling the odorants contained in the inspired air and giving us our appreciation of foods and perfumes, etc. The trigeminal nerves provide the sensations of touch, pain, hot, cold and itch, and also the sensation of nasal airflow perceived as a cool sensation on inspiration. The trigeminal nerves are important in detecting the presence of pollutants such as ammonia, sulphur dioxide, ozone and a range of organic substances, such as menthol, acetone, and pyridine (Doty, 1975).

Chemical or physical stimuli to the nasal epithelium may initiate potent respiratory and cardiovascular reflexes via stimulation of trigeminal nerves, resulting in expiration with apnoea, closure of the larynx, and bradycardia. Mild stimuli result in sneezing and nasal hypersecretion (Eccles, 1982). These reflex responses protect the lower airways from inhalation of physical and chemical irritants. Sneezing may be initiated by a number of factors such as mechanical stimulation of the nasal epithelium, cooling of the skin, bright light in the eyes, irritation of the scalp near the frontal hairline, challenge with allergen extract, and by psychogenic causes (Eccles, 1982; Leung and Robson, 1994).

The trigeminal nerves in the nasal epithelium initiate the sneezing and hypersecretion associated with chemical and mechanical stimulation of the nasal epithelium, and with upper respiratory tract infection and allergy. The trigeminal nerves may also be responsible for neurogenic inflammation associated with nasal infection and allergy, as various inflammatory mediators have been found in these nerves (Woodhead, 1994). The nasal epithelium is innervated by both sympathetic and parasympathetic nerve fibres, which act as the efferent arms of autonomic nasal reflexes involving the nasal glands and blood vessels. The parasympathetic fibres supply the nasal glands and the sympathetic fibres control nasal blood flow and the filling of venous erectile tissue.

3. Effects of Pollutants on the Nose

The effects of air pollutants on the nose are diverse and complex as they are not only dependent on the nature and concentration of the pollutant, but also on the duration of the period of exposure. The situation may be further complicated by the presence of a mixture of pollutants and the presence of infectious and allergic diseases of the nose. It is difficult to relate the laboratory studies on healthy volunteers who may be exposed to a single pollutant for a short period, to the real life situation where there may be chronic exposure to a wide range of air pollutants. It is beyond the scope of this chapter to look at all the the effects of air pollutants on the nose in both healthy volunteers and patients with nasal disease. Instead, I will discuss in general terms how pollutants exert their effects on the nose.

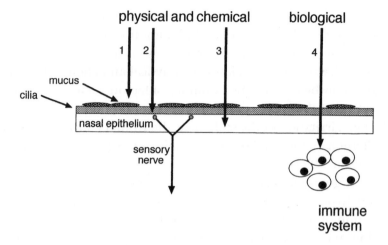

Fig. 3.   Effects of air pollution on the nose. Air pollutants exert their effects on the nose by physical, chemical and biological interactions with the nasal epithelium. The physical and chemical interactions affect: 1. mucociliary clearance 2. sensory nerves 3. epithelial cells. The biological interactions are with leukocytes within the nasal epithelium and include activation of the immune system and inflammation.

The effects of pollutants on the nose may be divided into physical, chemical and biological effects as illustrated in Fig. 3.

The physical effects of pollutants include effects of particulate matter on mucociliary clearance, where the deposition of large amounts of dust within the nose may overwhelm the capacity of mucociliary clearance and cause physical damage to epithelial cells and the stimulation of nasal sensory nerves. The chemical effects of pollutants include changes in the pH of nasal fluid and chemical reactions with cellular enzymes, structural proteins, and DNA. The biological effects of pollutants involve the immune system where the pollutants may act as adjuvants for allergic responses, or as antigens which trigger an allergic reaction.

3.1. *Effects on Sensory Nerves*

As previously mentioned above, the sensory nerves supplying the nasal cavity consist of the olfactory nerves and branches of the trigeminal nerves which are responsible for the perception of environmental chemicals. The olfactory receptors are located in the olfactory epithelium at the top of the back of the nasal cavity, whereas trigeminal nerve endings are distributed throughout the nasal epithelium. It is generally believed that chemical stimulation of the olfactory receptors leads to an odor sensation, whereas chemical stimulation of trigeminal nerve endings leads to a sensation of irritation (Silver, 1992). However, the trigeminal system serves more than just the sensation of irritation, as the cool sensation of nasal airflow is mediated by trigeminal nerves and there may be complex interactions between olfactory and trigeminal sensations to give the overall sensory impact of a chemical stimulus to the nose.

In considering the detection of air pollutants by the nose, it is probable that both the olfactory and trigeminal systems are involved. Low concentrations of air pollutants may give a sensation of an odor, and with increasing concentration, there will be a sensation of irritation. The trigeminal system acts as a defender at the entrance to the respiratory system and with increasing concentrations of a pollutant, there will be graded responses, i.e. low concentrations of pollutant cause nasal irritation which may cause nasal stuffiness and nasal congestion, and perhaps lead to other non specific complaints such as headache; higher concentrations that will result in reflex sneezing, nasal secretion and tearing of the eye; and with very high concentrations, there may be the initiation of respiratory inhibition and a slowing of breathing and periods of apnoea (Eccles, 1982; Angell-James and De Burgh-Daly, 1969).

The effects of acute exposure to pollutants such as sneezing and nasal secretion can be explained as respiratory reflexes which form an important component of respiratory defence, by preventing or limiting the exposure of the lungs to irritant pollutants. This type of reflex response could be initiated by both particulate and gaseous air pollutants. Chronic exposure to low levels of pollutant may have quite different effects which may be difficult to relate to any specific pollutant such as nasal stuffiness, headache and lethargy which are often associated with indoor pollutants and the so called "sick building syndrome" (Chester, 1993).

The interaction of pollutants with trigeminal sensory nerves is associated with other effects, apart from a sensation of irritation,

reflex sneezing and secretion. The trigeminal nerves also partici-
pate in the so called "axon reflex" and neurogenic inflammation,
which can give rise to nasal inflammation and nasal hyperreactivity
with symptoms of rhinitis. The mechanisms involved in neurogenic
inflammation and nasal hyperreactivity are illustrated in Fig. 4.

Pollutants stimulate trigeminal nerve endings in the nasal epithelium to initiate irritation and nasal reflexes, and these responses are
accompanied by local release of peptides from the nerve endings such
as substance P. The peptides released from sensory nerve endings are
known as tachykinins and they are believed to mediate neurogenic
inflammation and airway hyperreactivity (Maggi, 1993). Exposure to
pollutants, such as ozone, may cause neurogenic inflammation and
nasal hyperreactivity by causing the release of substance P, followed by
the release of histamine and the generation of prostaglandins (Koto
et al., 1995). Substance P, histamine and prostaglandins have a wide
range of pro inflammatory actions which will lead to nasal congestion,

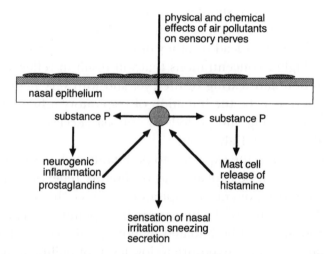

Fig. 4.   Trigeminal nerve axon reflex and nasal hyperreactivity. Air pollutants stimulate nasal trigeminal sensory nerves by physical and chemical actions to cause a
sensation of nasal irritation and protective nasal reflexes such as sneeze and nasal
secretion. The trigeminal nerve endings release substance P which initiates neurogenic inflammation and the release of histamine from Mast cells. Prostaglandins
and histamine interact with trigeminal nerve endings to cause a condition of nasal
hyperreactivity.

sneezing, nasal secretion and itching. Histamine and prostaglandins may also influence the sensitivity of the trigeminal nerve endings to increase their sensitivity to stimuli such as cold air and initiate a condition of hyperreactivity. Chronic exposure to pollutants such as ozone may cause rhinitis with hyperreactivity to the otherwise innocuous stimuli such as cold air and perfumes etc.

3.2. *Effects on Mucociliary Clearance*

Studies on air pollutants have demonstrated that a wide variety of pollutants such as grain dust, tobacco smoke, sulphur dioxide, cadmium, nickel, etc. cause a decrease in the rate of mucociliary clearance (Leopold, 1992; Holt, 1996). It is not clear whether the slowing of mucociliary clearance is caused by a slowing of ciliary beat frequency, or some effect on nasal mucus secretion, or a change in the depth or composition of the periciliary fluid. Cigarette smoke and sulphur dioxide may have direct effects on cilia, whereas heavy metals such as cadmium and nickel may influence the metabolism of epithelial cells and the availability of ATP for the energy required for the beating of cilia (Leopold, 1992; Riechelmann *et al.*, 1994).

3.3. *Effects on Epithelial Cells*

Pollutants may overwhelm nasal mucociliary clearance and cause physical and chemical damage to nasal epithelial cells. Septal perforations are seen in individuals exposed to arsenic and acids in the air, and carcinomas of the nose and paranasal sinuses have been linked to employment in the wood, leather and nickel industries (Leopold, 1994). Chronic exposure to pollutants may result in a condition of chronic inflammation and this will predispose to carcinoma by stimulating a more rapid turnover of nasal epithelial cells, and by exposing cells to oxidative damage as part of the inflammatory process.

3.4. *Effects on Immune System*

Pollutant dusts may contain biologically active materials such as allergens, bacteria, bacterial endotoxins and fungi. Chronic exposure to allergens may result in allergic rhinitis, such as seasonal or perennial allergic rhinitis associated with pollen or house dust mite allergens. Exposure to dust in industrial situations, such as grain dust, may result in a specific IgE response in sensitive individuals (Leopold, 1994). Some pollutants such as cigarette smoke and fibre glass have been shown to be non antigenic. However, it is possible that pollutants which do not have antigenic activity may influence the nasal immune response. Diesel exhaust particles may act as an adjuvant for the production of IgE antibody and provide a link between industrial pollution and allergic rhinitis (Muranaka *et al.*, 1986; Takafuji *et al.*, 1987). Even if pollutants do not act as adjuvants, they may increase the incidence of allergic rhinitis by causing a chronic inflammation of the nasal epithelium and causing an increased presence of leukocytes, which may predispose to inappropriate immune responses against harmless antigens such as pollen.

The natural defence mechanism of mucociliary clearance may be overwhelmed by high concentrations of dust in the environment, and if the dust particles contain bacteria or bacterial endotoxins, then a systemic response of fever may result and there may be an increased incidence of bacterial rhinitis and sinusitis.

3.5. *Rhinitis and Air Pollution*

The nose has a great capacity to clean the inspired air even under extreme conditions of pollution with high concentrations of particulate matter and industrial gases. The deposition of particulate matter in the nose exposes the nasal epithelium to the risk of infection, and even though the nose is the most commonly infected part of the body, it has a great ability to resist infection. Infectious rhinitis associated with the familiar symptoms of common cold is probably the most common of human diseases, with most adults suffering one or two periods of symptomatic infection each year and children suffering between 7–10 bouts of symptoms each year (Johnston and Holgate, 1996). Allergic rhinitis also has a high incidence, with incidence rates in Europe quoted as between 6–31% (Smith, 1999).

There has been much debate as to whether or not there has been an increase in allergic diseases of the airway, such as asthma and allergic rhinitis, in the last 20 years and on the role of air pollution in allergic airway disease (Wuthrich, 1989). It is now generally accepted that there has been an increase in the incidence of nasal allergy and a study in Australia has reported an increased incidence of 22% for seasonal allergic rhinitis between the period 1981 and 1990 (Smith, 1999). Whether the increased incidence of allergic rhinitis is due to changes in reporting methods or related to pollution or a decrease in incidence of infectious disease, is still controversial.

There is no doubt that acute exposure to high concentrations of air pollutants causes nasal responses such as nasal irritation, sneezing, nasal secretions, etc. as part of a non specific nasal defence response. However, it is much more difficult to determine the role of chronic or intermittent exposure to low levels of air pollutants in the development of nasal allergy and susceptibility to nasal infection. It is believed by some that chronic exposure to air pollutants may predispose to the development of allergic disease, but this picture is complicated by changes in the incidence of infectious diseases such as tuberculosis, which may also have an impact on the incidence of allergic disease (Cookson and Moffatt, 1997; Shirakawa *et al.*, 1997).

4. Summary

The nose acts as an air conditioner to condition the inspired air prior to gas exchange in the lungs and a major portion of inhaled dusts and pollutant gases are removed from the inspired air during its passage through the nose. Although the nasal epithelium is remarkably resistant to the injurious effects of the inspired air, exposure to air pollutants may result in nasal inflammation and rhinitis. A slowing of the rate of mucociliary clearance is a common effect of air pollutants and this may be predisposed to injury, infectious and allergic diseases.

References

Andersen I. and Molhave L. (1982) The ambient air. In *The Nose, Upper Airways Physiology and the Atmospheric Environment*, eds. Proctor D.F. and Andersen I. Elsevier, Amsterdam, pp. 307–336.

Angell-James J.E. and De Burgh-Daly M. (1969) Section of laryngology — Nasal reflexes. *Proc Roy Soc Med* **62**: 1287–1293.

Chester A.C. (1993) Hypothesis: The nasal fatigue reflex. *Integr Physiol Behav Sci* **28**: 76–83.

Cole P. (1982a) Upper respiratory airflow. In *The Nose, Upper Airways Physiology and the Atmospheric Environment*, eds. Proctor D.F. and Andersen I. Elsevier, Amsterdam, pp. 163–189.

Cole P. (1982b) Modification of inspired air. In *The Nose, Upper Airways Physiology and the Atmospheric Environment*, eds. Proctor D.F. and Andersen I. Elsevier, Amsterdam, pp. 351–376.

Cookson W. and Moffatt M.F. (1997) Asthma: An epidemic in the absence of infection? *Science* **275**: 41–42.

Cross C.E., Van d.V.A., Oneill C.A., Louie S. and Halliwell B. (1994) Oxidants, antioxidants, and respiratory tract lining fluids. *Environ Health Persp* **102**: 185–191.

Doty R.L. (1975) Intranasal trigeminal detection of chemical vapors by humans. *Physiol Behav* **14**: 855–859.

Eccles R. (1982) Neurological and pharmacological considerations. In *The Nose, Upper Airways Physiology and the Atmospheric Environment*, eds. Proctor D.F. and Andersen I. Elsevier, Amsterdam, pp. 191–214.

Eccles R. (1983) Physiology of nasal secretion. *Eur J Resp Dis* **62**: 115–119.

Grevers G. (1993) The role of fenestrated vessels for the secretory process in the nasal mucosa: A histological and transmission electron microscopic study in the rabit. *Laryngoscope* **103**: 1255–1258.

Holt G.R. (1996) Effects of air pollution on the upper aerodigestive tract. *Otolaryngology-Head Neck Surg* **114**: 201–204.

Housley D.G., Mudway I., Kelly F.J., Eccles R. and Richards R.J. (1995) Depletion of urate in human nasal lavage following in-vitro ozone exposure. *Int J Biochem Cell Biol* **27**: 1153–1159.

Johnston S. and Holgate S. (1996) Epidemiology of viral respiratory infections. In *Viral and Other Infections of the Human Respiratory Tract*, eds. Myint S. and Taylor-Robinson D. Chapman & Hall, London, pp. 1–38.

Koto H., Aizawa H., Takata S., Inoue H. and Hara N. (1995) An important role of tachykinins in ozone-induced airway hyperresponsiveness. *Am J Resp Crit Care Med* **151**: 1763–1769.

Kuo H.P., Rohde J.A.L., Tokuyama K., Barnes P.J. and Rogers D.F. (1990) Capsaicin and sensory neuropeptide stimulation of goblet cell secretion in guinea-pig trachea. *J Physiol* **431**: 629–641.

Leopold D.A. (1992) Pollution — the nose and sinuses. *Otolaryngology-Head Neck Surg* **106**: 713–719.

Leopold D.A. (1994) Nasal toxicity — end-points of concern in humans. *Inhal Toxicol* **6**: 23–39.

Leung A.K.C. and Robson W.L.M. (1994) Sneezing. *J Otolaryngol* **23**: 125–129.

Maggi C.A. (1993) Tachykinin receptors and airway pathophysiology. *Eur Resp J* **6**: 735–742.

Moriaty B.G., Robson A.M., Smallman L.A. and Drake-Lee A.B. (1991) Nasal mucociliary function: Comparison of saccharin clearance with ciliary beat frequency. *Rhinology* **29**: 173–179.

Muranaka M., Suzuki S., Koizumi K., Takafuji S., Miyamoto T., Ikemori R. and Tokiwa H. (1986) Adjuvant activity of diesel-exhaust particulates for the production of IgE antibody in mice. *J Allergy Clin Immunol* **77**: 616–623.

Persson C.G.A., Erjefalt I., Alkner U., Baumgarten C., Greiff L., Gustafsson B., Luts A., Pipkorn U., Sundler F., Svensson C. and Wollmer P. (1991) Plasma exudation as a first line respiratory mucosal defence. *Clin Exp Allergy* **21**: 17–24.

Proctor D.F. (1982) The mucociliary system. In *The Nose Upper Airway Physiology and the Atmospheric Environment*, eds. Proctor D.F. and Andersen I. Elsevier Biomedical Press, Amsterdam, pp. 245–278.

Riechelmann H., Kienast K., Schellenberg J. and Mann W.J. (1994) An *in vitro* model to study effects of airborne pollutants on human ciliary activity. *Rhinology* **32**: 105–108.

Rogers D.F. (1994) Airway goblet cells: Responsive and adaptable front-line defenders. *Eur Resp J* **7**: 1690–1706.

Shirakawa T., Enomoto T., Shimazu S.I. and Hopkin J.M. (1997) The inverse association between tuberculin responses and atopic disorder. *Science* **275**: 77–79.

Silver W.L. (1992) Neural and Pharmacological basis for nasal irritation. *Annals NY Acad Sci* **641**: 152–163.

Smith J.M. (1999) Epidemiology. In *Rhinitis Mechanisms and Management*, eds. Naclerio R.M., Durham S.R. and Mygind N. Marcel Dekker, New York, pp. 29–44.

Takafuji S., Suzuki S., Koizumi K., Tadokoro K., Miyamoto T., Ikemori R. and Muranaka M. (1987) Diesel-exhaust particulates inoculated by the intranasal route have an adjuvant activity for IgE production in mice. *J Allergy Clin Immunol* **79**: 639–645.

Wheatley J.R., Amis T.C. and Engel L.A. (1991) Nasal and oral airway pressure-flow relationships. *J Appl Physiol* **71**: 2317–2324.

Witek T.J. (1993) The nose as a target for adverse-effects from the environment — Applying advances in nasal physiological measurements and mechanisms. *Am J Ind Med* **24**: 649–657.

Woodhead C.J. (1994) Neuropeptides in nasal mucosa. *Clin Otolaryngol* **19**: 277–286.

Wuthrich B. (1989) Epidemiology of the allergic diseases: Are they really on the increase. *Int Arch Allergy Appl Immunol* **90**: 3–10.

CHAPTER 2

CARDIOVASCULAR EFFECTS OF PARTICLES

Helen C. Routledge and Jon G. Ayres

1. Introduction

That air pollution exerts health effects is now an accepted fact and is no longer a source of surprise. However, one remarkable finding that has arisen from the vast amount of research into this area over the last decade or so is that patients with cardiovascular disease may be those that are most at risk from inhaling polluted air. Time series studies, which model the relationship between day-to-day levels of air pollutants and health endpoints, have consistently demonstrated an association between both all-cause mortality and hospital admissions and ambient levels of a range of pollutants. This association has been observed between cities with different sources of pollution, climates and population structures in many different countries. The effects are mostly seen in the elderly and individuals with chronic illness. Meta-analysis of the available data, involving rigorous re-examination of the statistical methods employed, has confirmed that the observed increases in mortality are independent of the effects of confounding factors. On average, for every $10 \, \mu g/m^3$ rise in PM_{10}, there is an increase of about 1% in cardiovascular mortality on a day-to-day basis (Schwartz, 1994).

Despite the wealth of epidemiological data supporting this relationship, a plausible biological mechanism was needed. While it is intuitively logical that air pollution can affect patients with pulmonary disease, a mechanism for an effect on patients with heart disease was not immediately apparent until two hypotheses were advanced in the mid 1990s. Work addressing these hypotheses has, in addition to providing supportive evidence for both, also informed on identification of the specific pollutant(s) responsible and the susceptible populations at risk. The causal pathway is now clearer although many questions remain.

2. Epidemiology

2.1. *Air Pollution and Mortality*

The association between air pollution and total daily mortality has been established by over 200 time series from geographically distinct areas (see Schwartz, 1994 and Dockery, 2001 for meta-analysis and review of the evidence). In Europe, the APHEA project (Air Pollution and Health, a European Approach) aimed to quantify the short-term health effects of air pollution using a common methodology to collect data from 15 European cities, with a total population exceeding 25 million (Katsouyanni *et al.*, 1995). In Western European cities, an increase of $10 \mu g/m^3$ in SO_2 (UK annual level: $20–66 \mu g/m^3$) was associated with a 0.6% increase in daily all-cause mortality, the corresponding figure for PM_{10} being 0.4% (Katsouyanni *et al.*, 1997). Similar effects on all-cause mortality were demonstrated in the U.S. 20 Cities Study (Samet *et al.*, 2000). The estimated increase in the relative rate of death from all causes, in a population of more than 50 million, was 0.51% for each increase in the PM_{10} level of $10 \mu g/m^3$.

2.2. *Air Pollution and Cardiovascular Mortality and Morbidity*

Mortality

A significant proportion of total mortality in the western world is attributable to cardiovascular disease, where ischaemic heart disease is the leading cause of mortality in men over the age of 45 and in women over the age of 65. Consequently, knowing that air pollution was associated with all-cause mortality, it was logical to consider whether this effect was mediated in part through cardiac disease.

A number of time series studies have specifically considered the relationships between mortality from cardiovascular and respiratory causes and increases in ambient pollutant levels (Table 1). These data suggest that although the relative risks for pollution related deaths

Table 1.　Summary of time series studies of air pollution effects on mortality.

Time Series Study	Geography	Pollutants	Mortality Effect
Wichmann 1985	West Germany 1985	SO_2 TSP	8% ↑ mortality during smog 6% ↑ CVS mortality (15%↑ Admissions)
Schwartz 1990	London 1958–1972	Black Smoke SO_2	Significant predictors of all cause mortality
Katsouyanni 1990	Athens 1975–1982	SO_2 Black Smoke	Higher respiratory and CVS mortality on polluted days
Kinney 1991	Los Angeles County 1970–1979	Particles CO & NO_2	Strongly associated with daily CVS mortality
Schwartz 1992	Philadelphia 1973–1980	SO_2 TSP	5%↑ mortality/100 μg ↑SO_2 7%↑ mortality/100 μg ↑TSP 10%↑ CVS mortality
Pope 1992	Utah 1985–1989	PM_{10}	16%↑ mortality/100 μg ↑ PM_{10}
Dockery 1992	St Louis 1985–1986	PM_{10}	16%↑ mortality/100 μg ↑PM_{10}
Dockery 1993	6 U.S. Cities	Fine Particles Sulphates	Association between mortality and pollution level in city
Schwartz 1994	Meta-analysis	TSP	RR death =1.06 for 100 μg increase in TSP
Anderson 1996	London 1987–1992	Black Smoke SO_2 Ozone	2.5%↑ daily mortality/↑ 7–19 μg/m³ SO_2 also significant 3.6%↑ CVS mortality/ ↑7–36 ppb
Verhoeff 1996	Amsterdam 1986–1992	Black Smoke	RR mortality 1.19 for ↑100 μg/m³

Table 1.   (*Continued*)

Time Series Study	Geography	Pollutants	Mortality Effect
		PM_{10}	RR mortality 1.06 for $\uparrow 100\,\mu g/m^3$
		SO_2 CO	No consistent association
		Ozone	Positively associated w/ mortality
Katsouyanni 1997	12 European Cities 1991–1994 (APHEA)	PM_{10} SO_2	2% $\uparrow$ mortality/50 $\mu g/m^3$ 3% $\uparrow$ mortality/50 $\mu g/m^3$
Borja-Aburto 1997	Mexico City 1990–1992	TSP	Excess mortality 6%/$\uparrow 100\,\mu g/m^3$
Ponka 1998	Helsinki 1987–1993	PM_{10}	4.1% $\uparrow$ CVS mortality/$\uparrow 10\,\mu g/m^3$
		Ozone	9.9% $\uparrow$ CVS mortality/$\uparrow 20\,\mu g/m^3$
		NO_2	Additive effect w/PM_{10} and Ozone
Ostro 1999	Bangkok 1992–1995	PM_{10}	2% $\uparrow$ CVS mortality/$10\,\mu g/m^3$ $\uparrow$
Samet 2000	20 U.S.Cities 1987–1994	PM_{10}	$\uparrow$ rate of CVS/Resp mortality 0.68% for each $\uparrow PM_{10}$ of $10\,\mu g/m^3$
		(SO_2, CO, Ozone NO_2)	Weak associations
Roemer 2001	Amsterdam 1987–1998	Black Smoke	RR mortality 1.38 for $\uparrow 100\,\mu g/m^3$
		NO_2	RR mortality 1.10 for $\uparrow 100\,\mu g/m^3$
Kwon 2001	Seoul 1994–1998	$PM_{10}, SO_2,$	RR mortality 1.014/IQR$\uparrow$ PM_{10}
		CO, Ozone NO_2	RR mortality 1.020/IQR$\uparrow$ CO Effect 2.5–4.1% higher in CCF
Katsouyanni 2001	29 European Cities APHEA 2	PM_{10}	$\uparrow$ rate of CVS/Resp mortality 0.6% for each $\uparrow PM_{10}$ of $10\,\mu g/m^3$ Effect size greater in elderly; w/high NO_2 or in cold climates

are greater for respiratory than for cardiovascular causes, because of the size of the population at risk, the actual numbers of deaths are greater for cardiovascular diseases (Dockery, 2001).

In addition to the time series, survival analysis data derived from cohort studies of groups at high risk of cardiovascular mortality add further weight to the evidence for a cardiotoxic effect of air pollutants. Goldberg, for example, described daily mortality increasing linearly, as concentration of ambient particles increased, for individuals who had coronary artery disease and congestive heart failure (Goldberg *et al.*, 2001). Data describing the consequences of interventions leading to changes in the composition of ambient pollutants have also confirmed that decreases in both particulate matter and sulphur dioxide are associated with both immediate and long-term cardiovascular health benefits. Following a ban on coal sales within the city of Dublin in September 1990, Clancy and colleagues found a reduction in annual cardiovascular death rates of 10.3%, associated with a reduction in black smoke concentration of 35.6 $\mu g/m^3$ (Clancy *et al.*, 2002). In Hong Kong, a restriction introduced over one weekend, which required all power plants and vehicles to convert to low sulphur fuels, led to an immediate decline in deaths from all causes of 2.1% and in deaths from cardiovascular causes of 2.0% (Hedley *et al.*, 2002). There is also supporting evidence from the occupational setting, in that individuals who are involved in occupational exposure to particles have an increased risk of coronary artery disease (Sjogren, 1997).

Thus, the relationships between cardiovascular mortality and air pollution have been repeatedly demonstrated. The precise causes of these deaths, however, have been more difficult to determine. The majority of time series studies describe effects according to broad categories, relying on retrospective analysis of routine coding for both admissions and mortality. In the smog episode in Germany in 1985, deaths and admissions were more accurately coded on the basis of the international classification of diseases (ICD-9) for 94% of the cases (Wichmann *et al.*, 1989). Deaths due to heart failure, myocardial infarction and stroke were all increased significantly in the polluted areas, compared with the control areas. In this study, these increases were even more pronounced than those due to respiratory diseases.

More recently, Hoek *et al.* studied associations between daily variations in air pollution and specific cardiovascular causes of death in the Netherlands over 8 years. Effect estimates were calculated for 1 to 99 percentile increases in each pollutant, for particles equivalent to a rise of $80\,\mu g/m^3$ in 7 day mean PM_{10}. Effects were significant for total cardiovascular mortality (RR mortality: 1.012 for PM_{10}, 1.029 for SO_2, 1.055 for O_3), myocardial infarction and other ischaemic heart disease death (RR mortality 1.005 for PM_{10}, 1.015 for SO_2, 1.026 for O_3), but were most pronounced (3 times higher for all pollutants except ozone) for deaths from heart failure and arrhythmia (Hoek *et al.*, 2001).

Hospital admissions

Similar conclusions can be drawn from data on hospital admissions for cardiovascular disease (Table 2). The second phase of the APHEA project used pooled data from eight European cities and found a 1.1% rise in cardiac admissions for all ages, and a 1.3% rise in cardiac admissions over 65 years for a $10\,\mu g/m^3$ rise in PM_{10} (Le Tertre *et al.*, 2002). In the UK, findings from a London time series analysis were consistent with 1 in 50 myocardial infarctions treated at London hospitals being triggered by outdoor air pollution (Poloniecki *et al.*, 1997). A systematic review of the data, prepared for COMEAP (The Committee on the Medical Effects of Air Pollutants, UK Department of Health), estimated that a $10\,\mu g/m^3$ reduction in 24-hour average PM_{10} concentration would be associated with a 0.8% reduction in cardiovascular admissions (Anderson and Atkinson, 2001). Thus, across the UK, high levels of ambient pollution may be responsible for at least 6000 cardiovascular admissions per year (Poloniecki *et al.*, 1997). The specific relationship between air pollution and myocardial infarction has recently been strengthened by the findings of the Determinants of Myocardial Infarction Onset Study (Peters *et al.*, 2001). This multi-centre case-crossover investigation suggested that transient elevation in the concentration of fine particles (increase of $25\,\mu g/m^3$ $PM_{2.5}$), at levels still below current air quality standards, was associated with an increased risk (odds ratio 1.48) of myocardial infarction (MI) within 1 to 2 hours. In addition, high 24-hour concentrations of fine

Table 2.   Summary of time studies of air pollution effects on hospital admissions.

Time Series Study	Geography	Pollutants	Effect on Admissions
Schwartz 1995	Michigan 1986–1989	PM_{10} CO*	↑ Ischaemic heart disease admissions (RR 1.018 IQR↑ PM_{10}) and with heart failure (RR 1.024/ IQR↑PM_{10} and 1.022/IQR↑CO*)
Burnett 1995	Ontario 1983–1988	Particulate Sulphates	2.8% ↑ CVS admission/13 µg/m³ ↑
Morris 1995	7 U.S. Cities 1986–1989	CO	↑ Heart failure admissions (RR 1.10-1.37/10ppm↑ CO
Wordley 1997	Birmingham, UK 1992–1994	PM_{10}	↑ Risk of respiratory (2.4%) or cerebrovascular (2.1%) admission for 10 µg/m³ ↑ PM_{10}
Schwartz 1997	Tuscon 1997	PM_{10} CO Ozone/SO_2	2.75%↑CVS admission/ IQR↑ PM_{10} 2.79%↑CVS admission/ IQR↑ CO Little association
Burnett 1997	10 Canadian Cities 1981–1991	CO	RR Heart Failure admission 1.065/IQR ↑CO
Burnett 1997	Toronto 1992–1994	Ozone NO_2 SO_2	13% ↑ CVS admissions/IQR ↑ gaseous pollutants
Schwartz 1999	Eight U.S. Counties 1988–1990	PM_{10} CO	2.48% ↑ CVS admission/IQR ↑ 2.79% ↑ CVS admission/IQR ↑

particles were also associated with an elevated risk (odds ratio 1.69) of MI. The results at the two separate time periods were independent and additive, suggesting the possibility of two, possibly independent mechanisms.

Arrhythmias

In 1985, German smog related arrhythmia admissions were increased by 50% compared with the periods before and after the smog (Wichmann *et al.*, 1989). A panel study carried out by Peters *et al* adds further weight to the hypothesis that an increase in cardiac arrhythmia contributes to the rise in mortality associated with increases in ambient pollution levels (Peters *et al.*, 2000). In 100 patients with implantable cardioverter defibrillators in Boston USA, episodes of defibrillation were related to daily air pollution. The frequency of defibrillator discharges showed a significant correlation with increased levels of PM_{10} and $PM_{2.5}$, with a lag time of 2 days and an association with NO_2 levels on the previous day. In a sub-group of patients who had had at least 10 interventions to treat ventricular arrhythmia, the odds of a discharge tripled with an increase in NO_2 from the 5th to the 95th percentile, and increased by 60% for the equivalent rise in $PM_{2.5}$.

2.3. *Pollutants Implicated in Cardiovascular Health Effects*

While fine and ultrafine particles, predominantly derived from fossil fuel combustion, have been most strongly and consistently associated with cardiac mortality, questions still surround the importance of the major gaseous air pollutants. There is considerable evidence that levels of sulphur dioxide (SO_2) are associated with both mortality and admissions for cardiovascular disease (see Tables 1 and 2). In the Michigan study, for example, an increase in SO_2 of 18 ppb (interquartile rise) was associated with a RR of 1.014 in ischaemic heart disease admissions. In a number of studies, however, the mortality effect of SO_2 becomes insignificant after controlling for particulate matter (Schwartz and Morris, 1995; Schwartz and Dockery, 1992). Nitrogen dioxide (NO_2), carbon monoxide (CO) and ozone (O_3) have all been associated in time series analyses (see Tables 1 and 2) with cardiovascular mortality and admissions. It remains to be determined whether NO_2 and CO, both of which are good markers of vehicle generated pollution, are acting as the primary agents or are merely surrogate markers for another pollutant. If the latter the most likely is another metric for particles such as particle numbers or surface area.

3. Potential Mechanisms

In order to show that these associations are causal, plausible mechanisms of action are required. Evidence is accumulating in support of two possibly interlinked mechanisms by which low concentrations of pollutants in inspired air could have acute adverse cardiovascular effects:

(1) *Inhalation and interstitialisation* of fine particles might provoke an inflammatory response in the lungs, with the consequent release into the circulation of pro-thrombotic and inflammatory cytokines. A systemic acute-phase response of this nature would put individuals with coronary atheroma at increased risk of plaque rupture and thrombosis.

(2) *Cardiac autonomic control* may be affected by exposure to particulate matter or gaseous pollutants, leading to an increased risk of arrhythmia in susceptible patients.

3.1. *The Inflammatory Hypothesis*

A systemic inflammatory response to particulate air pollution was initially suggested in 1995 by Seaton, who postulated that such a response might precipitate acute coronary events as a result of an increase in blood coagulability (Seaton *et al.*, 1995). Since then, the relationships between systemic inflammation, the thrombophillic state and adverse coronary events in patients with coronary artery disease has become well established (Ferreiros, 1999; Biasucci, 1999).

The inflammatory theory of atherosclerosis

In the past, it was believed that atherosclerosis gradually and progressively led to the complete occlusion of an artery, thereby causing acute coronary events. We now understand that rupture of a non-stenotic but vulnerable atherosclerotic plaque leads to an acute coronary syndrome. The size of a plaque and its ability to cause stenosis and symptoms of angina bears no relation to its stability. Instead, plaques that are prone to rupture have characteristically histological features of a thin fibrous cap, numerous inflammatory cells and a substantial lipid core. Physical disruption of such a plaque allows circulating coagulation factors to come into contact with thrombogenic material in the lipid core, thereby instigating the formation of a potentially occluding thrombus. Much evidence now implicates inflammation with accumulation of activated mononuclear cells in the thinning of the fibrous cap and the disruption of the vulnerable atherosclerotic plaque. Inflammation within the plaque may result from accumulation of lipids, oxidant stress and infectious agents, or pro-inflammatory triggers from distant sites of infection and inflammation. Most recent research has focused on means of reducing inflammation and thus stabilising plaques, and little attention has been paid to possible environmental stimuli that might increase inflammation and the likelihood of an acute coronary syndrome occurring.

Inflammation and thrombogenesis

Also, increasingly recognised is the contribution of inflammation to athero-thrombosis and the direct involvement of inflammatory cytokines in activation of the coagulation pathways. Thrombin generation is initiated by the complexing of tissue factor, expressed on the surface of monocytes and endothelial cells, with factor VII of the extrinsic pathway. The generation of thrombin then activates platelets in addition to causing formation of fibrin. Inflammatory cytokines, including tumour necrosis factor α and interleukin-1, stimulate release of tissue factor from monocytes and endothelial cells, thus facilitating thrombin generation. In addition, these cytokines impair fibrinolysis by provoking release of plasminogen activator inhibitor and thrombin-activatable fibrinolysis inhibitor and reducing concentrations of activated protein C complexes. Within the complex biochemical chain of events occurring during clot formation, the coagulation pathway in turn activates inflammatory mediators. Activated factor X of the common pathway, for example, stimulates the synthesis and release of interleukins-6 and 8 (Becker, 2002). Thus, it can be seen that any external influence resulting in increases in circulating inflammatory cytokines may not only increase the risk of plaque rupture occurring, but also help to initiate and perpetuate the resulting thrombosis.

Epidemiological evidence for a systemic inflammatory response to air pollutants

In keeping with the above, increases in circulating markers of systemic inflammation have been associated with the risk of coronary events and cardiac death in observational studies. Elevated levels of C-reactive protein (CRP) predict risk of instability and death, not only in patients with stable angina and unstable angina, but also in asymptomatic individuals (Biasucci, 1999; Zebrack *et al.*, 2002). Analysis of stored blood samples from the subjects recruited for large epidemiological studies for other reasons has revealed evidence for a systemic inflammatory response caused by exposure to air pollutants. Increases in CRP and plasma viscosity (determined largely by plasma fibrinogen concentration, which is also a marker of cardiovascular risk) occurred in association with high levels of particulate pollution in studies involving nearly 4000 healthy adults (Peters *et al.*, 1997; Peters *et al.*, 2001). During an air pollution episode which occurred during the period of study, the odds of observing CRP concentrations above the 90th percentile increased 3-fold, and the odds ratio for plasma viscosity above the 95th percentile of the distribution was 3.6 in men and 2.3 in women (Peters *et al.*, 2001). However, this does not necessarily mean that the same effect would occur in populations chronically exposed to lower levels of the same pollutants.

Initiation of the inflammatory response

Following these epidemiological observations, experimental work began to investigate how a systemic inflammatory response might be initiated and amplified following pollutant exposure. Circulating acute phase proteins such as CRP are produced by hepatocytes, and plasma viscosity is dependent on levels of plasma proteins such as fibrinogen that increase with inflammation. Increased expression of the genes coding for acute-phase proteins is driven by cytokines such as interleukin-6, which are produced by activated macrophages and other blood mononuclear cells.

In vitro work and animal exposure studies have demonstrated that this sequence of events might well be triggered by pulmonary injury in response to air pollutants. Fine particles are capable of penetrating the alveolar epithelium (Donaldson and MacNee, 1998), where they may cause local inflammation and oxidative stress by several mechanisms, such as direct toxicity to lung cells, stimulation of alveolar macrophages to release reactive oxygen metabolites and stimulation of alveolar macrophages to secrete cytokines which recruit polymorphonuclear cells causing further damage (Donaldson, 2000). Rats exposed to particulate matter *in vivo* develop significant pulmonary injury, as evidenced by increases in broncho-alveolar lavage fluid neutrophils and lymphocytes, and by histological assessment of lung tissue (Dye *et al.*, 2001). Human alveolar epithelial cells, exposed to combustion-derived particles *in vitro* (albeit at high concentrations), released pro-inflammatory cytokines such as IL-6, IL-8 and TNF-alpha (Veronesi *et al.*, 1999; Jimenez *et al.*, 2002). Cytokine secretion in these cell models is preceded by activation of the redox-sensitive transcription factor nuclear factor kappa B (Kennedy *et al.*, 1998; Shukla *et al.*, 2000) and is inhibited by the free radical scavenger N-acetyl-L-cysteine (Quay *et al.*, 1998).

Confirmation of these findings in humans has been provided by Salvi and colleagues (Salvi *et al.*, 1999), who exposed 15 healthy volunteers to diesel exhaust ($[PM_{10}]$:300 $\mu g/m^3$, $[NO_2]$: 1.6 ppm, $[CO]$: 7.5 ppm) for one hour and found an increase in inflammatory cells in both broncho-alveolar lavage and bronchial biopsies, when compared with air exposure in the same subjects. Six hours after diesel exposure, there was a significant increase in neutrophils, mast cells, T lymphocytes and upregulation of the endothelial adhesion molecules ICAM-1 and VCAM (implicated in the recruitment of leukocytes), when compared with air or NO_2 exposure alone. However, these findings can also be interpreted as NO_2 exerting an adjuvant effect on the inflammatory response, suggested to be due to particles. Diesel exhaust also enhanced gene transcription of cytokines and chemokines in bronchial tissue (Salvi *et al.*, 2000).

In animals, ambient PM samples collected and then administered by intra-tracheal instillation have enabled closer investigation of the specific properties of airborne particles that may be responsible for causing these local inflammatory responses (Costa and Dreher, 1997). The degree of oxidative stress and the release of cytokines have now repeatedly been found to be related to size, surface area and to the transition metal content of particles (Frampton *et al.*, 1999; Ghio *et al.*, 2000). Recently, using a rat model of short-term exposure to concentrated ambient particles, significant oxidative stress was demonstrated by *in situ* chemiluminescence in both the lung and the heart. Increases in oxidant levels were also triggered by residual oil fly ash particles but not by carbon black aerosols alone, suggesting that the carbon core of the ambient aerosol is not an active contributor to inflammation (Gurgueira *et al.*, 2002). Increased lung oxidant generation was associated with the transition metal content of the exposure, notably iron, manganese, copper and zinc; whilst in the heart, inhalation of particles containing aluminium, silicon and titanium were most closely associated with oxidant production (Gurgueira *et al.*, 2002).

Experimental evidence for generation of a systemic inflammatory response following air pollution exposure

Work in animals has suggested that following induction of mild pulmonary inflammation by repeated exposure to particles, increased rates of production and release of polymorphonuclear leukocytes from the bone marrow into the peripheral blood soon occur (Mukae *et al.*, 2001). The magnitude of these changes was related to the percentage of alveolar macrophages containing particles. Instillation of supernatants from human alveolar macrophages that had been incubated with PM_{10} into rabbit lungs, induced similar changes in the animals' bone marrow. This systemic inflammatory response was not seen after instillation of supernatant from unstimulated macrophages (Mukae *et al.*, 2000).

Following their controlled human diesel exhaust exposures, Salvi and colleagues found significant increases in neutrophils in the peripheral blood at 6 hours (Salvi *et al.*, 1999), demonstrating that acute short-term diesel exhaust exposure produces pulmonary inflammation, followed by a well-defined and marked systemic inflammatory response. Together with the animal data, these results would suggest that inhalation of particles leads to release of cytokines from inflammatory cells in the lung, which in turn stimulate release of neutrophils from the bone marrow and their transit from blood back to the airway tissues. Acute exposure to diesel exhaust was also associated with significant thrombocytosis (Salvi *et al.*, 1999), another marker of the acute phase response, and in a similar protocol, Delvin and colleagues found that exposure to concentrated ambient particles produced mild pulmonary inflammation, followed by increases in plasma fibrinogen (Ghio *et al.*, 2000). To date, controlled human exposure studies have not been undertaken to confirm an acute rise in CRP or plasma viscosity, in response to specific pollutants.

Cardiovascular consequences of the inflammatory response to air pollutants

Although direct evidence is not yet available in humans, this inflammatory response to particulate pollutants might well result in both destabilisation of atherosclerotic plaques and induction of thrombogenesis. Rabbits exposed to particulate pollution showed a systemic inflammatory response with increases in circulating polymorphonuclear leucocytes and evidence of bone marrow stimulation. In keeping with the above hypothesis atherosclerotic plaques in these PM_{10}, exposed animals were found to show more characteristics of instability when compared with plaques in the sham exposed group (thin plaque caps, presence of inflammatory cells, fewer smooth muscle cells) (Suwa *et al.*, 2002). Coronary thrombosis, in direct response to inhaled pollutants, is more difficult to demonstrate experimentally and indirect evidence of a pro-coagulant state relying on circulating fibrinogen concentration has failed to provide conclusive evidence. In a 2-year cross-sectional survey in London data on concentrations of plasma fibrinogen for over 7000 office workers were combined with air pollution data. An increase in the 24-hour mean NO_2 or CO concentration during the previous day from the 10th to the 90th percentile was associated with a 1.5% higher fibrinogen concentration (Pekkanen *et al.*, 2000). Since then, Ghio and colleagues found increases in circulating fibrinogen, following chamber exposure to concentrated ambient particles (Ghio *et al.*, 2000), but in a third study, blood samples taken over 18 months from 112 subjects revealed a negative correlation between ambient particle measurements and levels of fibrinogen (Seaton *et al.*, 1999). Fibrinogen concentrations have previously been found to be negatively related to environmental temperatures (Stout and Crawford, 1991) and this is likely to have a significant impact on the results of such observational studies.

Particles in the circulation

While most attention has focused on the assumption that local pulmonary inflammation following pollution exposure is the sole trigger of the observed systemic inflammatory response, an alternative hypothesis is that ultrafine particles themselves can cross the alveolo-capillary barrier and pass into the pulmonary circulation. This has been demonstrated with 40 nanometre fluorescent polystyrene beads in isolated perfused rabbit lungs (Delaunois *et al.*, 1999), while ultrafine (5–10 nanometre) carbon particles radio-labelled with [99m]Technetium have been found to pass into the systemic circulation in five healthy humans following inhalation. Radioactivity was detected in the blood after one minute and reached a maximum between 10 and 20 minutes with substantial radioactivity over the liver and other areas of the body (Nemmar *et al.*, 2002). Accumulation in the liver, perhaps by Kupffer cells, suggests that inflammation in response to pollution could be initiated at extra-pulmonary sites. Oxidative stress is known to increase the permeability of epithelial cells (Lay *et al.*, 2001) and this would increase the likelihood of not only the cytokine signals, but also the particles themselves of entering the circulation.

3.2. The Autonomic Hypothesis

Epidemiological data highlights an association between cardiac arrhythmia and levels of ambient pollutants in the preceding days. Although myocardial ischaemia and acute coronary events may often be the trigger of ventricular arrhythmia, whether air pollutants may themselves exert a direct effect on cardiac rhythm or not, has not been completely understood.

Epidemiological evidence for disturbance in cardiac autonomic control in response to exposure to air pollution

Disturbances in the control of heart rate and rhythm, in response to particulate pollution, were originally suggested by two large observational studies. During an air pollution episode in Central Europe in January 1985, which resulted in an elevated number of hospital admissions for cardiovascular diseases, resting heart rates in nearly 3000 subjects were increased during the pollution episode, compared with control periods (in men: +1.75 bpm, {0.43, 3.07} in women: +2.87 bpm {1.42, 4.32} mean change {95% CI}) (Peters *et al.*, 1999). In addition, when concentrations of suspended particles and sulphur dioxide were considered as continuous variables throughout the whole study period, this association remained even after adjusting for cardiovascular risk factors and meteorological parameters (Peters *et al.*, 1999). In a panel study in Utah in the winter of 1995 and 1996, oxygen saturation and heart rate using pulse-oximetry were measured daily in 90 elderly subjects (Pope *et al.*, 1999). While there was no evidence of pollution related hypoxia, pulse rate and the odds of the pulse rate being elevated by 5 or 10 beats per minute were associated with PM_{10} on the previous 1 to 5 days.

An increase in resting heart rate suggests an alteration in autonomic control of the heart and has long been recognised as an independent risk factor for total cardiovascular mortality, myocardial infarction and sudden death (Dyer *et al.*, 1980; Hjalmarson *et al.*, 1990). Increases in the heart rate have been seen to precede ventricular arrhythmia in patients whose rhythms are monitored by implantable defibrillator devices (Nemec *et al.*, 1999). The observational studies outlined above have thus suggested a plausible link between exposure to particulate pollution and sudden cardiac death in susceptible individuals.

Cardiac autonomic control, heart rate variability and mortality

Analysis of heart rate variability in large cohorts of healthy subjects and those with hypertension, ischaemic heart disease and hypertension has confirmed that impaired cardiac vagal control is a powerful and independent predictor of mortality. Heart rate variability (HRV) measurement is a non-invasive technique used to quantify cardiac autonomic control. The principle behind the technique is that variability in rate is not a property intrinsic to the heart, but is instead determined by the action of the cardiac autonomic nervous system on the sinus node. The vagus nerve exerts a dominant inhibitory influence on resting heart rate (Katona *et al.*, 1982) and fires phasically at a frequency that corresponds with the respiratory rate. The resulting oscillation in the heart rate, known as respiratory sinus arrhythmia, constitutes the majority of HR variability. Measurement of beat-to-beat changes in heart periodicity, i.e. the degree of "high frequency" variability, thus reflects vagal influence on the heart (Task Force, 1996). Standardised techniques are used to obtain a series of RR intervals from ECG recordings, i.e. the time intervals between consecutive normal beats. From these recordings, taken either over short periods with controlled respiration or over 24 hours using Holter monitoring, are derived a number of measures of variability both in the time and in the frequency domains. The standard deviation of RR interval differences (SDNN) is a simple statistical measure which quantifies overall variability, resulting from the influence of predominantly the vagus, but also of the sympathetic nervous system. RMSSD, the root mean square of successive RR interval differences and the high frequency power (derived from power spectral analysis using the Fast Fourier transformation) solely reflect vagal influence. Normal ranges are available for both healthy individuals of all ages and for those with cardiovascular disease.

Decreased heart rate variability occurs in patients with established heart diseases such as myocardial infarction (Lombardi *et al.*, 1996) and chronic heart failure, shown to be an independent predictor of cardiac death (La Rovere *et al.*, 1998; Nolan *et al.*, 1998). The ATRAMI investigators who studied 1284 survivors of a recent myocardial infarction, found low values of HRV to be associated with a 2-year mortality of 10% compared with 2% when HRV was preserved. Further analysis of these mortality data revealed specific associations between depressed HRV, sudden death and sustained ventricular tachycardia (La Rovere *et al.*, 2001). Low HRV has also been demonstrated to be a risk factor for adverse cardiac events in apparently healthy subjects enrolled in the Framingham study (Tsuji *et al.*, 1996). These relationships between HRV and mortality are independent of conventional risk factors such as left ventricular function (La Rovere *et al.*, 1998). Possible mechanisms by which preserved cardiac vagal activity might beneficially influence prognosis include a decrease in myocardial oxygen demand, a reduction in sympathetic activity and a decreased susceptibility of the ventricular myocardium to lethal arrhythmia. There is strong animal evidence that increased sympathetic and reduced vagal control results in an increased susceptibility of ischaemic myocardium to ventricular fibrillation (Schwartz *et al.*, 1988).

Attempts to modify HRV with drugs and thereby improve prognosis have led to further understanding of some of the factors contributing to impaired cardiac autonomic control. Both angiotensin II and aldosterone have inhibitory effects on the cardiac vagus such that neurohormonal activation in heart failure is thought to be the cause of observed decreases in HRV. Environmental factors that may have a detrimental effect on cardiac autonomic control have only recently become the subject of investigation. The epidemiological evidence for an association between exposure to air pollutants, tachycardia and mortality from cardiac arrhythmia has led investigators to use non-invasive measures of cardiac autonomic control in a number of observational studies.

Observational studies of the association of pollution exposure to heart rate variability

In the first of these investigations, 7 elderly subjects underwent ambulatory ECG monitoring before, during and after particulate pollution episodes from a steel mill. After controlling for absolute heart rate, small consistent negative associations between pollution (PM_{10}) levels and same day measures of HRV (SDNN) were found (Pope *et al.*, 1999). In a further group of 26 elderly men (mean age 81), over a three-week period, the risk of an individual having low heart rate variability (SDNN, HF power) was significantly increased on days when $PM_{2.5}$ levels were high. The largest inverse associations were found for individuals with pre-existing cardiovascular disease (Liao *et al.*, 1999). In Boston, 21 subjects (aged 53–87) were observed intermittently over a period of 4 months with ambulatory ECG monitoring. Interquartile increases in $PM_{2.5}$ and ozone resulted in a combined effect equivalent to a 33% reduction in the mean RMSSD (Gold *et al.*, 2000).

In an occupational setting, Magari and colleagues addressed one of the limitations to these earlier studies (Magari *et al.*, 2001). Previously, estimation of personal exposure to pollutants had relied on data obtained from regional monitoring stations. Magari used personal exposure monitors in a cohort of 40 boilermakers, who wore 24-hour ambulatory ECG monitors at home and in the work place. In addition, this method allowed more accurate estimation of the time course of any observed effect. In these young industrial workers, half of whom were current smokers, a significant negative association was found between 4-hour $PM_{2.5}$ exposure (increases of $100\,\mu g/m^3$) and 5-minute measures of SDNN. This effect appeared to be biphasic with a short acting component (several minutes) and a longer effect over several hours. However, personal $PM_{2.5}$ levels were higher (mean $167\,\mu g/m^3 \pm$ S.D $320\,\mu g/m^3$) than ambient levels typically reported in Boston and there were differences in activity levels during and away from work, which make interpretation of alterations in HRV measures difficult.

Experimental evidence for adverse effects of air pollution on cardiac autonomic control

Experimental exposure studies in this area are limited. Rats with pulmonary hypertension exposed to particulate matter showed a dose-related increase in incidence and duration of serious arrhythmia, with no preceding hypoxia (Watkinson *et al.*, 1998). In a series of studies using dogs with partially ligated coronary arteries, exposure to concentrated ambient particles via tracheostomy caused a rise in heart rate, rising with increasing PM_{10} exposure as well as alterations in HRV measures of cardiac autonomic control (Godleski et al., 2000). Experimental laboratory exposure to SO_2 in humans has also recently been shown to exert significant adverse effects on HRV (Tunnicliffe et al., 2001).

Potential mechanisms for the effect of pollutants on the cardiac autonomic nervous system

How inhalation of pollutants and in particular fine particles might exert adverse effects on the cardiac autonomic nervous system remains to be fully elucidated. In keeping with the inflammatory hypothesis, inhaled particles may indirectly promote an autonomic stress response as a result of cytokine release. Alternatively, a direct neural effect might be attributable to stimulation of naso-pharyngeal, upper or lower airway receptors. Animal work has demonstrated that stimulation of "rapidly acting receptors" (RARs) can mediate powerful neural influences on the cardiovascular system (Yeates and Mauderly, 2001). RARs occur throughout the respiratory tract from the nose to the bronchi and are characterised by a rapid adaptation to a mechanical stimulus. They also respond, in a more prolonged manner, to a variety of chemical stimuli or irritants, including sulphur dioxide, smoke, dusts and inflammatory mediators (Widdicombe, 2001). The response to inhaled substances differs according to the location of the receptor (Nishino et al., 1996) and between individuals, and may also depend on the amount of mucus being secreted (Sant'Ambrogio and Widdicombe, 2001). Respiratory reflexes, such as cough and bronchoconstriction, arising from afferent receptors in the larynx and upper airways will in turn influence arterial blood pressure and heart rate. Impulses from irritant receptors in the airways are transmitted via the vagal nerves and are centrally processed in the medulla with consequent cardiovascular effects, including a parasympathetically mediated bradycardia (Nishino et al., 1996). Thus, inhalation of an irritant to the upper respiratory tract can result in a reflex, the efferent component of which (or the resulting change in respiratory pattern) would exert an influence on the cardiac vagus nerve.

3.3. *Air Pollution and Coronary Vasoconstriction*

One final pathophysiological mechanism which might explain the epidemiological findings and which incorporates both of the above hypotheses, has recently been suggested by Brook and colleagues (Brook *et al.*, 2002). Using controlled exposures to concentrated ambient particles and ozone in combination, they demonstrated that short-term inhalation of pollutants altered vascular function in a manner that promotes cardiac events. Inhalation of particles and ozone for 2 hours caused significant brachial artery vasoconstriction, compared with filtered air. Coronary and brachial artery reactivity are strongly correlated and so such changes could promote ischaemia in individuals with underlying coronary artery disease. Observational evidence has, in addition, recently linked ambient pollutant exposure to increased risk of ECG ST segment depression, suggestive of myocardial ischaemia. In 45 individuals with coronary artery disease, undergoing bi-weekly exercise testing, the likelihood of a positive test was associated with higher levels of $PM_{2.5}$ (Pekkanen *et al.*, 2002). Potential biological mechanisms for pollutant induced coronary vasoconstriction include reflex increases in sympathetic nervous system activity as a result of stimulation of airway receptors, or an acute increase in vascular endothelin release as a result of systemic inflammation and cytokine release.

The four mechanistic hypotheses, inflammation, thrombosis, autonomic influence and arterial reactivity, might each independently, or perhaps more likely in combination, explain the observed association between air pollution and both cardiovascular morbidity and mortality (Fig. 1). For example, in a susceptible individual with coronary artery disease, exposure to pollution might cause systemic inflammation, increasing the likelihood of plaque rupture. In addition, any adverse influence on cardiac autonomic control, particularly in an individual in whom it is already impaired, would then increase the vulnerability of the acutely ischaemic or failing myocardium to lethal ventricular arrhythmia (Zareba *et al.*, 2001).

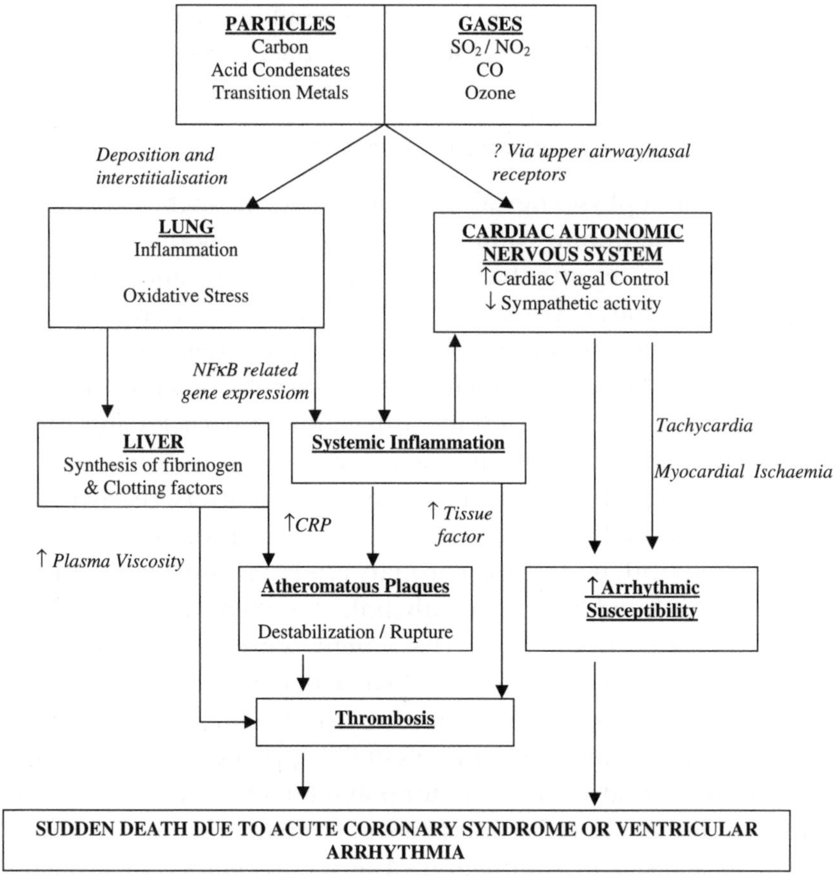

Fig. 1.

Short-term increases in morbidity and mortality from heart failure might also be explained by a combination of arrhythmic deaths, repeated ischaemic insults or impaired cardiac autonomic control, leading to tachycardia and hence worsening ventricular function.

4. Future Experimental Research and Considerations in Exposure Studies

The mechanistic pathways by which both particulate and gaseous air pollutants exert their undoubted adverse effects on the cardiovascular system are becoming clearer. There remain a number of unanswered questions to be addressed by ongoing experimental work and in particular by human exposure studies. Firstly, the epidemiological data have suggested that particular populations are at most risk. Considering the hypothetical pathways (Fig. 1), one might assume that those that are most prone to the local pulmonary inflammatory effect of inhaled pollutants would also be those that are most at risk of adverse cardiovascular outcomes. Current research is addressing the influence of chronic lung disease on the deposition of fine particles at differing levels of the respiratory tract. A clearer idea of where the particles are deposited and where they might be acting would help to define not only the population at risk, but also the size and nature of the particles/gases responsible. A related question to be answered in order to clarify potential autonomic influences, is whether particular pollutants reach airway receptors and what precise influence they have upon these receptors. A second group of patients at high risk according to this hypothesis would be those in whom cardiac autonomic control is already impaired, and this might well be addressed by cohort studies of patients with pre-existing cardiac disease.

Finally, the importance of chronic exposure to air pollutants in determining cardiovascular risk must also be addressed. While the majority of data available relates short-term changes in pollutant levels to acute changes in mortality, two large prospective cohort studies report that long-term exposure to fine particulate air pollution may have significant impacts on cardiovascular mortality (Dockery *et al.*, 1993; Pope *et al.*, 2002). Most recently, an 8-year study from the Netherlands addressed the issue of long-term exposure to traffic related pollutants and cardiopulmonary mortality. Hoek and colleagues found that living within 100 m of a main road, and hence being exposed to the highest levels of both black smoke and nitrogen dioxide, was associated with a relative risk of cardiopulmonary mortality of 1.95 (Hoek *et al.*, 2002). Clearly, the autonomic hypothesis is unlikely to play a role in explaining this long-term association, whilst a relationship between chronic exposure, low-level inflammation and atherogenesis is not unimaginable. In addition to the relationship between coronary plaque rupture and inflammatory stimuli, there is growing evidence of the importance of inflammation in the atherogenic process itself. In patients undergoing diagnostic coronary angiography, serological evidence of multiple exposure to infectious agents (e.g. chlamydia) is related to the extent of atherosclerosis and to long-term prognosis (Espinola-Klein *et al.*, 2002). Although this awaits supportive experimental evidence, one might hypothesise that long-term exposure to the components of traffic-related pollution, as described in the Netherlands study, might also be a stimulus to atherogenesis, thus explaining its association with increased mortality risk in the long term.

References

Anderson H.A. and Atkinson R.W. (2001) Association between ambient particles and daily admissions for cardiovascular diseases. Dept of Health, London.

Becker R.C. (2002) Antithrombotic therapy after myocardial infarction. *N Eng J Med* **347**: 1019–1022.

Biasucci L.L.G.(1999) Elevated levels of c-reactive protein at discharge in patients with unstable angina predict recurrent instability. *Circulation* **99**: 855–860.

Brook R.D., Brook J.R., Urch B., Vincent R., Rajagopalan S. and Silverman F. (2002) Inhalation of fine particulate air pollution and ozone causes acute arterial vasoconstriction in healthy adults. *Circulation* **105**: 1534–1536.

Clancy L., Goodman P., Sinclair H. and Dockery D.W. (2002) Effect of air-pollution control on death rates in Dublin, Ireland: An intervention study. *Lancet* **360**: 1210–1214.

Costa D.L. and Dreher K.L. (1997) Bioavailable transition metals in particulate matter mediate cardiopulmonary injury in healthy and compromised animal models. *Environ Health Perspect* **5**: 1053–1060.

Delaunois A.G.N., Nemery B., Nemmar A. and Gustin P. (1999) Can ultrafine particles cross the alveolo-capilliary border in isolated perfused rabbit lungs? *Am J Resp Crit Care Med* **159**: A30.

Dockery D.W. (2001) Epidemiologic evidence of cardiovascular effects of particulate air pollution. *Environ Health Perspect* **109**(Suppl 4): 483–486.

Dockery D.W., Pope A.C.d., Xu X., *et al.* (1993) An association between air pollution and mortality in six U.S. cities. *New Eng J Med* **329**: 1753–1759.

Donaldson K. (2000) Studies on the inflammatory potential of fine and ultrafine particles of carbon black, titanium dioxide and polystyrene/latex. *Am J Resp Crit Care Med* **161**: A 911.

Donaldson K.L.X. and MacNee W. (1998) Ultrafine (nanometre) particle mediated lung injury. *J Aerosol Sci* **29**: 553–560.

Dye J.A., Lehmann J.R., McGee J.K., *et al.* (2001) Acute pulmonary toxicity of particulate matter filter extracts in rats: Coherence with epidemiologic studies in Utah Valley residents. *Environ Health Perspect* **109**(Suppl 3): 395–403.

Dyer A.R., Persky V., Stamler J., *et al.* (1980) Heart rate as a prognostic factor for coronary heart disease and mortality: Findings in three Chicago epidemiologic studies. *Am J Epidemiol* **112**: 736–749.

Espinola-Klein C., Rupprecht H.J., Blankenberg S., *et al.* (2002) Impact of infectious burden on extent and long-term prognosis of atherosclerosis. *Circulation* **105**: 15–21.

Ferreiros E.B., C.P. (1999) Independant prognostic value of elevated c-reactive protein in unstable Angina. *Circulation* **100**: 1958–1963.

Frampton M.W., Ghio A.J., Samet J.M., Carson J.L., Carter J.D. and Devlin R.B. (1999) Effects of aqueous extracts of PM(10) filters from the Utah valley on human airway epithelial cells. *Am J Physiol* **277**: L960–L967.

Ghio A.J., Kim C. and Devlin R.B. (2000) Concentrated ambient air particles induce mild pulmonary inflammation in healthy human volunteers. *Am J Resp Crit Care Med* **162**: 981–988.

Ghio A.J., Richards J.H., Carter J.D. and Madden M.C. (2000) Accumulation of iron in the rat lung after tracheal instillation of diesel particles. *Toxicol Pathol* **28**: 619–627.

Godleski J.J., Verrier R.L., Koutrakis P., *et al.* (2000) Mechanisms of morbidity and mortality from exposure to ambient air particles. *Research Report – Health Effects Institute* 2000; 5–88.

Gold D.R., Litonjua A., Schwartz J., *et al.* (2000) Ambient pollution and heart rate variability. *Circulation* **101**: 1267–1273.

Goldberg M.S., Burnett R.T., Bailar J.C., 3rd, *et al.* (2001) Identification of persons with cardio-respiratory conditions who are at risk of dying from the acute effects of ambient air particles. *Environ Health Perspect* **109**(Suppl 4): 487–494.

Gurgueira S.A., Lawrence J., Coull B., Murthy G.G. and Gonzalez-Flecha B. (2002) Rapid increases in the steady-state concentration of reactive oxygen species in the lungs and heart after particulate air pollution inhalation. *Environ Health Perspect* **110**: 749–755.

Hedley A.J., Wong C.M., Thach T.Q., Ma S., Lam T.H. and Anderson H.R. (2002) Cardiorespiratory and all-cause mortality after restrictions on sulphur content of fuel in Hong Kong: An intervention study. *Lancet* **360**: 1646–1652.

Hjalmarson A.G., E.A. Kjekshus J., Schieman G., Nicod P., Henning H. and Ross J. Jr. (1990) Influence of heart rate on mortality after acute myocardial infarction. *Am J Cardiol* **65**: 547–553.

Hoek G., Brunekreef B., Fischer P. and van Wijnen J. (2001) The association between air pollution and heart failure, arrhythmia, embolism, thrombosis, and other cardiovascular causes of death in a time series study. *Epidemiology* **12**: 355–357.

Hoek G., Brunekreef B., Goldbohm S., Fischer P. and van den Brandt P.A. (2002) Association between mortality and indicators of traffic-related air pollution in the Netherlands: A cohort study. *Lancet* **360**: 1203–1209.

Jimenez L.A., Drost E.M., Gilmour P.S., Rahman I., Antonicelli F. and Ritchie H. (2002) PM(10)-exposed macrophages stimulate a proinflammatory response in lung epithelial cells via TNF-alpha. *Am J Physiol Lung Cell Mol Physiol* **282**: L237–L248.

Katona P.G., McLean M., Dighton D.H. and Guz A. (1982) Sympathetic and parasympathetic cardiac control in athletes and nonathletes at rest. *J Appl Physiol* **52**: 1652–1657.

Katsouyanni K., Touloumi G., Spix C., *et al.* (1997) Short-term effects of ambient sulphur dioxide and particulate matter on mortality in 12 European cities: Results from time series data from the APHEA project. Air Pollution and Health: A European Approach. *BMJ* **314**: 1658–1663.

Katsouyanni K., Zmirou D., Spix C., *et al.* (1995) Short-term effects of air pollution on health: A European approach using epidemiological time-series data. The APHEA project: Background, objectives, design. *Eur Resp J* **8**: 1030–1038.

Kennedy T., Ghio A.J., Reed W., *et al.* (1998) Copper-dependent inflammation and nuclear factor-kappaB activation by particulate air pollution. *Am J Resp Cell Mol Biol* **19**: 366–378.

La Rovere M., Bigger J.T., Jr., Marcus F.I., Mortara A., Schwartz P.J. (1998) Baroreflex sensitivity and heart-rate variability in prediction of total cardiac mortality after myocardial infarction. ATRAMI (Autonomic Tone and Reflexes After Myocardial Infarction) Investigators. *Lancet* **351**: 478–484.

La Rovere M.T., Pinna G.D., Hohnloser S.H., *et al.* (2001) Baroreflex sensitivity and heart rate variability in the identification of patients at risk for life-threatening arrhythmias: Implications for clinical trials. *Circulation* **103**: 2072–2077.

Lay J.C., Zeman K.L., Ghio A.J. and Bennett W.D. (2001) Effects of inhaled iron oxide particles on alveolar epithelial permeability in normal subjects. *Inhal Toxicol* **13**: 1065–1078.

Le Tertre A., Medina S., Samoli E., *et al.* (2002) Short-term effects of particulate air pollution on cardiovascular diseases in eight European cities. *J Epidemiol Commun Health* **56**: 773–779.

Liao D., Creason J., Shy C., Williams R., Watts R. and Zweidinger R. (1999) Daily variation of particulate air pollution and poor cardiac autonomic control in the elderly. *Environ Health Perspec* **107**: 521–525.

Lombardi F., Sandrone G., Spinnler M.T., *et al.* (1996) Heart rate variability in the early hours of an acute myocardial infarction. *Am J Cardiol* **77**: 1037–1044.

Magari S.R., Hauser R., Schwartz J., Williams P.L., Smith T.J. and Christiani D.C. (2001) Association of heart rate variability with occupational and environmental exposure to particulate air pollution. *Circulation* **104**: 986–991.

Mukae H., Hogg J.C., English D., Vincent R. and van Eeden S.F. (2000) Phagocytosis of particulate air pollutants by human alveolar macrophages stimulates the bone marrow. *Am J Physiol Lung Cell Mol Physiol* **279**: L924–L931.

Mukae H., Vincent R., Quinlan K., *et al.* (2001) The effect of repeated exposure to particulate air pollution (PM10) on the bone marrow. *Am J Resp Crit Care Med* **163**: 201–209.

Nemec J., Hammill S.C. and Shen W.K. (1999) Increase in heart rate precedes episodes of ventricular tachycardia and ventricular fibrillation in patients with implantable cardioverter defibrillators: Analysis of spontaneous ventricular tachycardia database. *Pacing Clin Electrophysiol* **22**: 1729–1738.

Nemmar A., Hoet P.H., Vanquickenborne B., *et al.* (2002) Passage of inhaled particles into the blood circulation in humans. *Circulation* **105**: 411–414.

Nishino T., Tagaito Y., Isono S. (1996) Cough and other reflexes on irritation of airway mucosa in man. *Pulm Pharmacol* **9**: 285–292.

Nolan J., Batin P.D., Andrews R., *et al.* (1998) Prospective study of heart rate variability and mortality in chronic heart failure: Results of the United Kingdom heart failure evaluation and assessment of risk trial (UK-heart). *Circulation* **98**: 1510–1516.

Pekkanen J., Brunner E.J., Anderson H.R., Tiittanen P. and Atkinson R.W. (2000) Daily concentrations of air pollution and plasma fibrinogen in London. *Occup Environ Med* **57**: 818–822.

Pekkanen J., Peters A., Hoek G., *et al.* (2002) Particulate air pollution and risk of ST-segment depression during repeated submaximal exercise tests among subjects with coronary heart disease: The Exposure and Risk Assessment for Fine and Ultrafine Particles in Ambient Air (ULTRA) study. *Circulation* **106**: 933–938.

Peters A., Dockery D.W., Muller J.E. and Mittleman M.A. (2001) Increased particulate air pollution and the triggering of myocardial infarction. *Circulation* **103**: 2810–2815.

Peters A., Doring A., Wichmann H.E. and Koenig W. (1997) Increased plasma viscosity during an air pollution episode: A link to mortality? *Lancet* **349**: 1582–1587.

Peters A., Frohlich M., Doring A., *et al.* (2001) Particulate air pollution is associated with an acute phase response in men; results from the MONICA-Augsburg Study. *Eur Heart J* **22**: 1198–1204.

Peters A., Liu E., Verrier R.L., *et al.* (2000) Air pollution and incidence of cardiac arrhythmia. *Epidemiology* **11**: 11–17.

Peters A., Perz S., Doring A., Stieber J., Koenig W. and Wichmann H.E. (1999) Increases in heart rate during an air pollution episode. *Am J Epidemiol* **150**: 1094–1098.

Poloniecki J.D., Atkinson R.W., de L.A.P. and Anderson H.R. (1997) Daily time series for cardiovascular hospital admissions and previous day's air pollution in London, UK. *Occup Environ Med* **54**: 535–540.

Pope C.A., 3rd, Burnett R.T., Thun M.J., *et al.* (2002) Lung cancer, cardiopulmonary mortality, and long-term exposure to fine particulate air pollution. *JAMA* **287**: 1132–1141.

Pope C.A., 3rd, Verrier R.L., Lovett E.G., *et al.* (1999) Heart rate variability associated with particulate air pollution. *Am Heart J* **138**: 890–899.

Pope C.A., Dockery D.W., Kanner R.E., Villegas G.M. and Schwartz J. (1999) Oxygen saturation, pulse rate, and particulate air pollution: A daily time-series panel study. *Am J Resp Crit Care Med* **159**: 365–372.

Quay J.L., Reed W., Samet J. and Devlin R.B. (1998) Air pollution particles induce IL-6 gene expression in human airway epithelial cells via NF-kappaB activation. *Am J Resp Cell Mol Biol* **19**: 98–106.

Salvi S., Blomberg A., Rudell B., *et al.* (1999) Acute inflammatory responses in the airways and peripheral blood after short-term exposure to diesel exhaust in healthy human volunteers. *Am J Resp Crit Care Med* **159**: 702–709.

Salvi S.S., Nordenhall C., Blomberg A., *et al.* (2000) Acute exposure to diesel exhaust increases IL-8 and GRO-alpha production in healthy human airways. *Am J Resp Crit Care Med* **161**: 550–507.

Samet J.M.D., Curriero F.C., Coursac I. and Zeger S.L. (2000) Fine Particulate Air Pollution and Mortality in 20 U.S. Cities 1987–1994. *New Eng J Med* **343**: 1742–1749.

Sant'Ambrogio G. and Widdicombe J. (2001) Reflexes from airway rapidly adapting receptors. *Resp Physiol* **125**: 33–45.

Schwartz J and Dockery D.W. (1992) Particulate air pollution and daily mortality in Steubenville, Ohio. *Am J Epidemiol* **135**: 12–19.

Schwartz J. (1994) Air pollution and daily mortality: A review and meta analysis. *Environ Res* **64:** 36–52.

Schwartz J. (1994) What are people dying of on high air pollution days? *Environ Res* **64:** 26–35.

Schwartz J. and Dockery D.W. (1992) Increased mortality in Philadelphia associated with daily air pollution concentrations. *Am Rev Resp Dis* **145**: 600–604.

Schwartz J. and Morris R. (1995) Air pollution and hospital admissions for cardiovascular disease in Detroit, Michigan. *Am J Epidemiol* **142**: 23–35.

Schwartz P., Vanoli E., Stramba-Badiale M., De F.G.M., Billman G.E. and Foreman RD. (1988) Autonomic mechanisms and sudden death. New insights from analysis of baroreceptor reflexes in conscious dogs with and without a myocardial infarction. *Circulation* **78**: 969–979.

Seaton A., MacNee W., Donaldson K. and Godden D. (1995) Particulate air pollution and acute health effects. *Lancet* **345**: 176–178.

Seaton A., Soutar A., Crawford V., *et al.* (1999) Particulate air pollution and the blood. *Thorax* **54**: 1027–1032.

Shukla A., Timblin C., BeruBe K., *et al.* (2000) Inhaled particulate matter causes expression of nuclear factor kappa B related genes and oxidant dependent NF kappa B activation *in vitro*. *Am J Resp Cell Mol Biol* **23**: 182–187.

Sjogren B. (1997) Occupational exposure to dust: Inflammation and ischaemic heart disease. *Occup Environ Med* **54**: 446–469.

Stout R.W. and Crawford V. (1991) Seasonal variations in fibrinogen concentrations among elderly people. *Lancet* **338**: 9–13.

Suwa T., Hogg J.C., Quinlan K.B., Ohgami A., Vincent R. and van Eeden S.F. (2002) Particulate air pollution induces progression of atherosclerosis. *J Am Coll Cardiol* **39**: 935–942.

Task Force. (1996) Heart rate variability: Standards of measurement, physiological interpretation and clinical use. Task Force of the European Society of Cardiology and the North American Society of Pacing and Electrophysiology. *Circulation* **93**: 1043–1065.

Tsuji H., Larson M.G., Venditti F.J., Jr., *et al.* (1996) Impact of reduced heart rate variability on risk for cardiac events. The Framingham Heart Study. *Circulation* **94**: 2850–2855.

Tunnicliffe W.S., Hilton M.F., Harrison R.M. and Ayres J.G. (2001) The effect of sulphur dioxide exposure on indices of heart rate variability in normal and asthmatic adults. *Eur Resp J* **17**: 604–608.

Veronesi B., Oortgiesen M., Carter J.D. and Devlin R.B. (1999) Particulate matter initiates inflammatory cytokine release by activation of capsaicin and acid receptors in a human bronchial epithelial cell line. *Toxicol Appl Pharmacol* **154**: 106–115.

Watkinson W.P., Campen M.J. and Costa D.L. (1998) Cardiac arrhythmia induction after exposure to residual oil fly ash particles in a rodent model of pulmonary hypertension. *Toxicol Sci* **41**: 209–216.

Wichmann H.E., Mueller W., Allhoff P., *et al.* (1989) Health effects during a smog episode in West Germany in 1985. *Environ Health Perspect* **79**: 89–99.

Widdicombe J. (2001) Airway receptors. *Resp Physiol* **125**: 3–15.

Yeates D.B. and Mauderly J.L. (2001) Inhaled environmental/occupational irritants and allergens: Mechanisms of cardiovascular and systemic responses. Introduction. *Environ Health Perspect* **109**(Suppl 4): 479–481.

Zareba W., Nomura A. and Couderc J.P. (2001) Cardiovascular effects of air pollution: what to measure in ECG? *Environ Health Perspect* **109**(Suppl 4): 533–538.

Zebrack J.S., Muhlestein J.B., Horne B.D. and Anderson J.L. (2002) The IHCSG. C-reactive protein and angiographic coronary artery disease: Independent and additive predictors of risk in subjects with angina. *J Am Coll Cardiol* **39**: 632–637.

CHAPTER 3

POINT SOURCES OF AIR POLLUTION — INVESTIGATION OF POSSIBLE HEALTH EFFECTS USING SMALL AREA METHODS

P. Elliott

1. Introduction

This chapter concerns the initial investigation of possible health effects related to a point source of air pollution, such as an industrial complex, a factory chimney or a municipal incinerator. Most often, the initial enquiry will assess the risk of disease, based on routinely available data, in an area in the immediate vicinity of the source, and compare it with that which is expected from national or regional rates, or the disease experience of a more distant area. Two types of enquiry can be considered: (i) investigations carried out because of *a priori* concerns about the potential health effects of a polluting source, and (ii) *post hoc* investigations carried out, following claims of disease excess in the vicinity (so-called "cluster" investigation).

Often, it is difficult to distinguish between these two types of investigation (Dolk *et al.*, 1977) because concerns about a raised disease incidence in an area can rapidly, by association, focus attention on one or more polluting sources in the area as possible causes. The difference between them is however important. While the first type of study falls under the traditional paradigm of hypothesis-led investigation, the second does not, since suggestion of excess disease risk in the area leads to the investigation being undertaken in the first place!

In the following sections, steps in the initial assessment of disease risk, in an area near a polluting source, are described, including issues of data availability and quality, confounding and possible biases. The problem of cluster investigation is also discussed. Where a disease excess is observed, usually confirmatory analyses in different areas with similarly polluting sources (if such can be found) and preferably in different time periods are required. In a well-known example of asthma epidemics in Barcelona, the fact that the epidemics were closely related in time to the loading and unloading of soya beans at the docks, allowed the probable cause of the epidemics to be identified and appropriate preventive action to be taken (Antó and Sunyer, 1992).

Further investigation of a disease excess in a particular locality, or associated with a specific source of pollution, will include a detailed understanding of possible routes of exposure, and possibly involve individual exposure assessment and/or biomarker studies, and the study of potential risk factors at individual level (i.e. case-control studies), including occupational and lifestyle factors such as smoking. These latter studies are beyond the scope of this chapter, but pertinent details can be found elsewhere in this volume.

2. Data Sources

We turn to the data needed for studies of potential health effects near point sources of air pollution. These include health data, population data (to enable risk estimates to be calculated), air pollution data and data on potentially confounding variables. As with all types of epidemiological enquiry, geographical (small-area) studies are subject to a number of problems related to the availability and quality of the data. Apparent local variations in disease could reflect differences between populations in completeness of ascertainment (e.g. in cancer registration (Best and Wakefield, 1999)), diagnostic accuracy, coding, hospital admissions policies and access for hospital data, and (for mortality) survival rates; or, if they depend on symptom reporting among potentially exposed and unexposed populations, the possibility of reporting biases must also be considered. Population estimates may be distorted by incomplete enumeration of the population (e.g. at census) or by recent migration (Arnold *et al.*, 1999). Such artefacts need to be considered in the interpretation of apparently raised risks in the vicinity of a pollution source.

In this chapter, these issues are illustrated with particular reference to the UK, where data availability including advent of geographic coding of health data, and statistical, computing and Geographic Information System (GIS) developments, have combined to enable the initial investigation of environment and health problems to be undertaken rapidly using routine data. Specifically, the UK has established a Small Area Health Statistics Unit (SAHSU) with the specific remit to:

(1) Examine quickly the reports of unusual clusters of disease, particularly in the neighbourhood of industrial installations.
(2) Build up reliable background information on the distribution of disease amongst small areas.
(3) Explore and develop methods for the study of the available statistics in order to detect reliably any unusual incidence of disease.
(4) Develop the methodology for analysing and interpreting statistics relating to small-areas.

SAHSU has developed a Rapid Inquiry Facility to enable statistics for the initial assessment of disease occurrence near a point source (or in a particular area) to be produced quickly based on routine data sources. This is further discussed in Sec. 3.1.

A similar system has been established in Finland, where, in common with other Nordic countries, linked data systems and geographic coding at individual level are available (Staines and Jarup, 2000). In many other countries including Italy, France and Germany, as well as Canada and the US, problems of data availability have so far limited the possibility of carrying out similar rapid analysis of routine data at a fine geographic scale. Nonetheless, geographic analysis can be done for larger geographic units such as commune in Italy (Clayton and Bernardinelli, 1992) or Département in France (Mollié, in press), as well as in purpose-designed studies (Goldberg *et al.*, 1999; Kanarek, 1980).

2.1. *Health Data*

In order to carry out small-area analyses of health statistics in the vicinity of a polluting source, geographic coding of the health data is required. In the UK, residential postcodes are used to locate individual health events. This offers high geographic resolution as there are currently around 2 million postcodes in the UK, approximately 14 households per postcode. The postcode "centroid" can be located as a point on a map to a 10–100 m precision. Recent work by the Ordnance Survey (Address Point) can locate each residential address nominally to +/− 0.1 m.

Availability of national routinely postcoded health and vital statistics data in England and Wales is summarised in Table 1. While births and all-cause mortality data are essentially complete, cause-specific mortality is subject to variability in diagnosis and possible coding artefacts. For cancer registration which is not statutory in the UK, under-ascertainment is a potential source of error, as is possible duplication.

Hospital episode data are a further resource for small area analysis in the UK. There are a number of problems with their routine use including diagnostic completeness and accuracy, variation in quality and completeness of the coding, and variable interpretation of the coding rules themselves. In England and Wales, the data are episodic rather than person based, although approximate linkages can be achieved using date of birth, sex and postcode. They have been used, for example, to examine the risk of admission for respiratory illness in children, in relation to the proximity of residence to the nearest main roads (Wilkinson *et al.*, 1999; Edwards *et al.*, 1994).

Congenital anomaly data held on the national registry (maintained for England and Wales by the Office for National Statistics) have generally high levels of under-ascertainment, but may be useful for

(1) Particular anomalies with higher levels of ascertainment, such as Down's syndrome and major neural tube defects, provided that information on terminations of these conditions is also available.

Table 1. Examples of national postcoded health and vital statistics data in England and Wales*.

Data	Year (from)	Source	Comment
Mortality	1981	ONS	Complete, but diagnostic accuracy and coding of underlying cause of death may vary.
Cancer incidence	1974	ONS	Various degrees of under-ascertainment and duplication, both between registries and at sub-regional level. The quality of the national register has improved in recent years.
Congenital anomalies	1983	ONS	Major problem of under-ascertainment in national register. Some specialised local registries have much higher levels of ascertainment.
Hospital Episode Statistics	1991	DoH Welsh Office	Huge database (ca. 10 million records/year in England). Episode, not person based. Diagnostic accuracy, coding etc. varies between hospitals.
Births	1981	ONS	Complete. Provides data on birth weight and postcoded denominator for early childhood events.
Stillbirths	1981	ONS	Data on stillbirths complete, but data on early and late abortions not routinely available.

*Some of these data are also available from local sources, e.g. Primary Care Trusts and regional cancer registries.
ONS   Office for National Statistics.
DoH   Department of Health (England).

(2) Localised analyses (e.g. near one or more point sources) where ascertainment rates may be relatively constant over a small area.

Other data potentially available for analysis include General Practitioner data, although currently not routinely available (except for samples of the population in anonymised databases), and local data from high quality computerised databases. The latter have been used, for example, in small area studies of asthma (Livingstone *et al.*, 1996).

Alternatively, questionnaire data have been obtained from residents in purpose-designed surveys. As already noted, such studies are liable to possible reporting biases, as residents living near to sources of pollution may be more likely to report symptoms than "control" populations, even in the absence of any health effect from environmental pollution. This potential for bias is illustrated by results of a study that investigated symptom reporting among residents living near a waste site containing chromium, compared with responses among a control population. While there was little overall difference in scores between the two communities on a general health questionnaire (SF-36), scores were lower among people living near the waste site, who believed that it was having an effect on their health (McCarron *et al.*, 2000). The authors interpreted this as reflecting the perception of harm and possible anxiety, rather than a health effect associated with toxicity from the site per se. Other examples where potential reporting biases may have been operating include studies of the health of residents living near coke works (Bhopal *et al.*, 1994), as well as asthma and wheeze reporting among children living close to main roads (Duhme *et al.*, 1996).

2.2. *Population Data*

In the UK, population data for small areas are available from the national census e.g. enumeration districts for 1991, and census output areas for 2001. A typical 1991 enumeration district gives population counts (by sex, in five-year age groups) and socio-economic data for about 400 people and enables appropriate standardisation to be carried out, i.e. calculation of a Standardised Mortality (or Morbidity) Ratio (SMR) by small area.

The census counts are themselves estimates. For instance, the "Estimating with Confidence" project in the UK provided adjustments of the raw 1991 census population statistics (Simpson *et al.*, 1995). Such work can provide valuable insights into the likely discrepancy between actual and estimated population sizes, as can local registers. For inter-censual years, population counts must not only take into account the usual demographic changes (e.g. births/deaths), but also migration as well. Population projections beyond the most recent census (and perhaps historically) will also often be required for small-area studies. In the future, computerised data from general practice will become an important subsidiary source of population data.

The frequent lack of a common geography between censuses introduces further error when a set of population counts by year is produced. In the UK, two-thirds of the censual enumeration districts changed between the 1981 and 1991 censuses, whilst the geographical units were again different in 1971 and 2001.

Although errors are likely to be small when populations are aggregated up to larger areas, this is not the case for small-area analyses. Potentially large errors in population estimation can be expected, for example, in areas of rapid development, or where there was substantial under-enumeration at census (e.g. for young single men in inner city areas) (Diamond, 1992). Where the total population size remains stable over time, nonetheless, there may have been substantial migration into and out of the area.

In the UK, event data can be linked to the population data via the postcode of residence, although in England and Wales, these links are only approximatations. In a small number of cases, postcodes themselves may be wrong or inaccurately located, or the postcode may be discontinued and later re-used. These sources of error in the population data introduce an additional degree of uncertainty to the estimates of disease risk.

2.3. *Exposure Assessment*

One of the key problems facing small-area analyses of health effects near a pollution source is that an estimate of population exposure to the pollutants of interest is often lacking. Where details of chimney stack height, operating conditions, meteorology and so forth are available, pollution modelling can give estimates of ambient air pollution concentrations in areas near the source which can then be fed into the statistical modelling of health risk. Ideally, such modelling should be supported by measured air pollution data either from fixed site sampling points, or preferably from personal sampling among a subset of the population. Appropriate data for pollution modelling may not be available, particularly if the concern is with historical exposures or perhaps cumulative exposures over many years. Again, these models take no account of travel and migration patterns, both through the study area during day-to-day activities, and into and out of the study region. Also, indoor and occupational exposures are ignored, insofar as they differ from outdoor exposures.

Given these difficulties of exposure estimation, resource has been made in the past to simple "distance-decline" models, with the often untested assumption that exposure, and hence risk, is greatest when it is nearest to the source; and with a decline in exposure levels and risk, when they are some distance from the source. Two possible models are illustrated in Fig. 1, the first with an exponential decline, and the second with a plateau near the source, followed by exponential decline.

Insofar as such simple models are likely to misclassify areas and the individuals who live within them, with respect to exposure to ambient air pollution, then any bias in such analyses is likely to be conservative, i.e. relative risk estimates are likely to be biased towards one (no association). Developments in the geographical coverage, quality and availability of environmental data, especially air pollution data, is leading to enhanced modelling of such exposures and their relation to the health data (Hodgson *et al.*, in press).

2.4. *Socioeconomic Confounding*

A major difficulty in the interpretation concerns the issue of confounding. This will arise when a third variable (the confounder) is both associated with the exposure of interest and with the health outcome, so that an apparent (non-causal) association of exposure

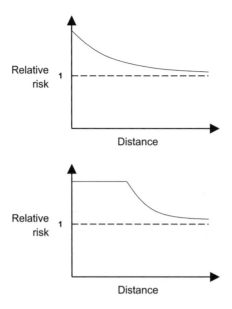

Fig. 1. Schematic representations of two simple modes of disease risk near a point source. Reproduced with permission of Arnold Publishers, *Stat Math Med Res* **41**: 137–159, 1995.

to disease is observed. Consider the plot shown in Fig. 2 where each dot represents one enumeration district near a municipal incinerator site in Great Britain. The abscissa gives distance in kilometres from the site, while the ordinate gives the value of a deprivation score for that enumeration district, based on census statistics (social class of head of household, overcrowding and unemployment). Higher scores define areas of greater deprivation (zero is the average score for Great Britain). The solid line gives the median deprivation score with distance. As can be seen, there is a trend of greater deprivation with proximity to the site. Consider also Fig. 3 which shows a range of diseases in different regions with a trend of increasing mortality at higher levels of deprivation (Eames *et al.*, 1993).

Taken together, the two figures show that the conditions for socio-economic confounding are fulfilled, with distance acting as a proxy for exposure to pollutants from the incinerator. All things being equal, we would expect to find higher than average rates of disease

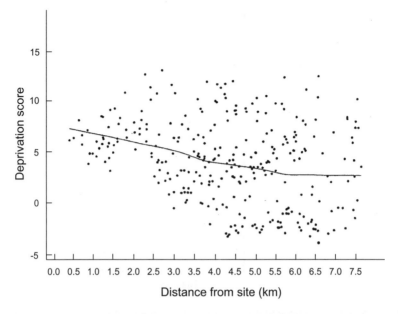

Fig. 2. Scatterplot of deprivation score with distance from a municipal incinerator. Reproduced with permission of BMJ Publishing Group, *J Epidemiol Commun Health* **49**(Suppl 2): 59–519, 1995.

near the incinerator, because of its socio-economic profile, irrespective of pollution in the vicinity.

Deprivation measures based on census statistics act merely as proxies for the complex mix of social, environmental and possibly genetic factors that may vary between areas. Ideally, we would wish to have direct measures of such variables at individual or small-area scale, in order to explore and account for the potential confounding. This is especially true of individual-level variables in the social environment that we know will powerfully affect the risk of disease, especially diet, alcohol drinking and smoking. Unfortunately, such data are rarely available with the exception of being collected as part of special surveys.

Since polluting sources may be located in socio-economically deprived areas, small-area studies of health risk in the vicinity of these plants need to take socio-economic confounding into account. For instance, a study investigating cancer risk near municipal solid waste incinerators in the UK found small excesses of lung, colon and

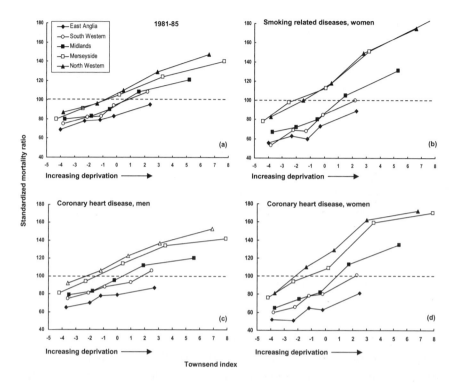

Fig. 3. Relationship of premature mortality from different causes in men and women by deprivations quantile for five health regions. Reproduced with permissions of the BMJ Publishing Group, *Br Med J* **307**: 1097–1102, 1993.

stomach cancers, which were also apparent before the incinerators were operational. Despite adjustment for socio-economic confounding in the analysis, it appears that residual confounding by socio-economic or other local factors was operating and explained the higher cancer risks in the vicinity of the plants (Elliott *et al.*, 1996).

3. Assessing Effects of Factory Emissions on the Health of Local Populations

This section addresses the investigation of health risk in the vicinity of a polluting source. Detailed accounts of the approach to such an investigation as well as the data analysis are available (Rothenberg and Thacker, 1992; Cartwright *et al.*, 1997). Key issues are summarised here. The steps involved in the *a priori* study of disease risk reading a polluting source include:

(1) Form a hypothesis.
(2) Select geographic region(s) and time period for study.
(3) Assemble and check the data.
(4) Obtain an estimate of risk.
(5) Write a report and feed back.
(6) End study or further investigation as indicated.

Investigation of a putative disease cluster, without a prior hypothesis, will be similar (steps 2 to 6). Such studies are further considered in Sec. 3.2 below. Each of these steps is now considered briefly.

Form a hypothesis

This will involve knowledge of the nature of the polluting source and the likely pollutants emitted. An understanding of their toxicology and possible health effects, and a review of previous studies around similar plants (if available) should enable the key health outcomes for study to be identified. It should be noted that studies with large numbers of end-points, possibly involving repeated analyses among several age-gender groups, will give rise to large numbers of statistical tests and the possibility that positive results will occur by chance alone (type I error).

Geographic regions and time period for study

It is important that the geographic scope and the time period of the study be identified at the outset to avoid the problem of "boundary shrinkage" which may accentuate estimates of disease risk, particularly in cluster investigation (see Sec. 3.2 below). Where air pollution data are available (usually from modelling), they can be used to inform the geographic extent of the study. If not, then arbitrary, distance bands around the source may be used. For example, the study of municipal solid waste incinerators mentioned above used a range of distances up to 7.5 km from each incinerator (Elliott *et al.*, 1996).

   Problems may arise in hilly terrain or where the local topography presents other natural boundaries to the dispersal of pollutants, since the distance approach, or pollution estimates based on Gaussian dispersion models, may give a poor reflection of pollution concentrations on the ground. Here, local monitoring to inform and validate the pollution models would be especially valuable, and undertaking purpose-designed surveys might need to be considered.

Assemble and check the data

Assembling the necessary health, population, confounder and air pollution data is a time-consuming process, especially if new data collection (e.g. symptom surveys) is required. Even if the study is to be based on routinely available data sources, obtaining and linking the data at the appropriate (high resolution) geographic scale may take several months. In the UK, as mentioned in Sec. 2, the Rapid Inquiry Facility of the Small Area Health Statistics Unit (SAHSU) can collate, analyse and report on the routine health statistics around any point in the country within a few days (Aylin *et al.*, 1999). An example is given in Table 2 and discussed in Sec. 3.1 below. Data checking is an essential step, as one or more of a number of errors that may seriously affect risk estimates can occur. Cases may be assigned to a "default" postcode (the treating hospital or local post office for example) and hence an apparent cluster be detected at that postcode. Cases may also be

Table 2. Populations, observed and expected counts and standardised mortality and morbidity ratios after standardisation for age, sex and deprivation from Rapid Inquiry Facility output.

Area	Population	Observed Cases	Expected Cases	Relative Risk*	95% CI
Mortality from respiratory diseases					
Within 2 km	71495	1196	1120.6	1.07	1.01–1.13
2–7.5 km	783943	13970	12765.8	1.09	1.08–1.11
Hospital admissions for respiratory diseases					
Within 2 km	71495	2834	2867.2	0.99	0.95–1.03
2–7.5 km	783943	30827	29239.7	1.05	1.04–1.07

*standardised mortality and morbidity ratios.
From: Aylin P, *et al. J Public Health Med* 1999; **21**: 289–298 (with permission).

misdiagnosed or mis-coded, located incorrectly, or possibly in duplicates (especially in the cancer registry), that could lead to spuriously elevated risk estimates; and errors in the denominator could lead to under- or over-estimation of risk.

Obtain an estimate of risk

Once the health data, population data, possible confounder data and air pollution data, where available, are in place, and data checks have been done, then an estimate of risk is required. Usually, the Standardised Mortality or Morbidity Ratio (SMR) is obtained by comparing the observed numbers of cases in areas near and more distant from the source, or in high and low pollution areas, with the numbers expected based on the age and gender distribution of the population, calculated using indirect standardisation. Standard disease rates for some comparison population are required, usually national or regional rates. It is preferable that standardisation by socio-economic factors be done to deal with the problem of potential socio-economic confounding. Aylin *et al.*, 1999 give details of the calculation of the SMR in an Appendix.

Write a report and feed back

It is essential that a careful record is kept throughout the investigation, including details of contacts with members of the public, industry, pressure groups, media, etc. The investigation should not be regarded as complete until the results are reported (usually by the local department of public health), and the results fed back to the local population, industry and other key players (Rothenberg and Thacker, 1992).

Further investigation

Often, a detailed review of the available cases, scrutiny of the population at risk, etc., will result in risk estimates that are close to one (despite the potential for bias in the selection of areas at high risk, as discussed in Sec. 3.2, below); and following the completion and presentation of the final report, the investigation will also come to an end. Where there is still an unexplained excess of risk, further investigation might be indicated. This might include further local studies, e.g., special surveys to examine symptoms, GP records (Bhopal *et al.*, 1994; Bhopal *et al.*, 1998), occupational histories (Elliott *et al.*, 1992), or the replication of the study in other areas (Dolk *et al.*, 1997; Elliott *et al.*, 1992).

3.1. *Example of a Point Source Investigation*

Results of a typical point source investigation that were presented to a local Department of Public Health (Aylin *et al.*, 1999), are summarised in Table 2. A member of the public had complained to their Member of Parliament concerning possible health effects of chemical air pollution near two factories on the same site in a deprived area. No changes in illness patterns had been noted by local GPs. A detailed report had been compiled by local environmental health officers who had inspected the site. Respiratory mortality was generally high in that part of the district, and the local Department of Public Health focused the investigation on respiratory admissions and mortality near the two factories. The coordinates for the two factories were passed on to the SAHSU Rapid Inquiry Facility.

After standardisation for age, sex and deprivation, mortality from respiratory disease appeared to be raised, although the excess was both seen within 2 km (RR 1.07, 95%CI 1.01–1.13) and more distant from the two factories (2–7.5 km; RR 1.09, 95%CI 1.08–1.11), suggesting that this might reflect generally higher rates than those of the standard region used for calculating expected values, rather than an excess associated specifically with the source. There was no excess of hospital admissions for respiratory illness < 2 km from the source (RR 0.99, 95% CI 0.95–1.03) although there was an apparent small excess at 2–7.5 km (RR 1.05, 95% CI 1.04–1.07). The excesses observed were all < 10%.

A report was provided to the referring department, giving details of the request, data used, time period and the geographic extent of the investigation, age and International Classification of Disease (ICD) groups studied, maps of the area including deprivation profile, results and brief commentary, including an outline of limitations of the analysis. This was used to inform the local Department of Public Health's report. No further action was deemed necessary.

3.2. *Cluster Investigation*

Cluster investigation is an area of work that is becoming increasingly prevalent and may implicate air pollution from local industry as a possible cause. A putative disease cluster may first be suspected by concerned members of the public, be reported by the media, or perhaps come to light following concerns about a pollution source in the vicinity, as discussed above. Note that as areas at apparent "low" risk do not come to the attention of the authorities, there is built-in bias towards reporting areas with disease excess.

For rare diseases in small areas, an apparent disease excess may depend crucially on only one or two cases, and these may not stand detailed scrutiny during an initial case-by-case review (Rothenberg and Thacker, 1992). The next few steps will usually involve identification of a geographic area and specification of a time frame so that a population at risk, and hence disease rates, can be calculated. These decisions can be crucial as apparent "clusters" may depend critically on the boundaries chosen in time or space, so-called "boundary shrinkage": "The more narrowly the underlying population is defined, the lesser will be the number of expected cases, the greater will be the estimate of the excess rate, and often the more pronounced will be the statistical significance" (Olsen *et al.*, 1996).

If the apparent "cluster" is subsequently linked to a pollution source, statistical testing is formally invalidated because of the post hoc nature of the observation. Only rarely have such investigations led to the identification of new or unsuspected causes of disease (Antó and Sunyer, 1992).

4. Conclusions

The study of the possible health effects from point sources of air pollution is not straight-forward and is subject to various pitfalls that can catch the unwary. Nonetheless, given current public, scientific and legislative concerns, there is a growing need for such analyses. Crucially, a number of datasets need to be assembled and integrated on a common geographic scale including health data, population data, air pollution exposure data, and socio-economic data, and the problems of availability, data quality, and errors in the geographic matching can lead to artefacts that could seriously bias the estimates of risk. Often, exposure data are sparse or unavailable, and use has been made of simple radial-dispersion models that may inadequately capture the true population exposure. Where resulting risk estimates show only a small excess, given all the problems of data quality, they may not be distinguishable from residual confounding by socio-economic or other factors, or bias.

Recent advances in computing, Geographic Information Systems (GIS) and the availability of high geographic-resolution health data, have enabled the initial investigation of point source exposures to be largely automated within a dedicated system, as has been developed in SAHSU for the UK, in Finland (National Institute of Public Health), Denmark and some other European countries (Aylin *et al.*, 2002). Where a disease excess is found in a particular locality, then pending data availability, the study can be replicated elsewhere, or in a different time period, from within such a system. This is particularly useful in "cluster" investigations, where geographic/temporal associations with local industry often do not reflect prior hypotheses, and for rare diseases, where small numbers may preclude statistically robust inference.

Increased availability of air pollution data at local scale, and advances in exposure modelling and personal sampling, should enable improved estimates of risk around point sources of air pollution to be obtained in the future.

Acknowledgements

The Small Area Health Statistics Unit is funded by a grant from the Department of Health, Department of the Environment, Food and Rural Affairs, Environment Agency, Scottish Executive, Welsh Assembly Government and the Northern Ireland Department of Health,

Social Services and Public Safety. The views expressed in this publication are those of the author and not necessarily that of the funding departments.

References

Antó J.M. and Sunyer J. (1992) In *Geographical and Environmental Epidemiology: Methods for Small-Area Studies*, eds. Elliott P., Cuzick J., English D. and Stern R. Oxford University Press, Oxford, pp. 323–341.

Arnold R., Wakefield J., Elliott P. and Quinn M., eds. (1999) *Population Counts in Small Areas: Implications for Studies of Environment and Health*. HMSO, London, *Studies in Medical and Population Subjects* 62.

Aylin P., *et al.* (2002) *Epidemiology* 13(4) (Suppl): S102.

Aylin P., *et al.* (1999) *J Publ Health Med* 21: 289–298.

Best N. and Wakefield J. (1999) *J Royal Stat Soc A* 162: 363–382.

Bhopal R.S., Phillimore P., Moffatt S. and Foy C. (1994) *J Epidemiol Community Health* 48: 237–247.

Bhopal R.S., *et al.* (1998) *Occup Environ Med* 55: 812–822.

Cartwright R., *et al. Handbook and Guide to the Investigation of Clusters of Diseases*. Leeds University Print Services, Leeds, pp. 120.

Clayton D. and Bernardinelli L. (1992) In *Geographical and Environmental Epidemiology: Methods for Small-Area Studies*, eds. Elliott P., Cuzick J., English D. and Stern R. Oxford University Press, Oxford, pp. 205–220.

Diamond I. (1992) In *Geographical and Environmental Epidemiology: Methods for Small-Area Studies*, eds. Elliott P., Cuzick J., English D. and Stern R. Oxford University Press, Oxford, pp. 96–105.

Dolk H., Elliott P., Shaddick G., Walls P. and Grundy C. (1997) *Am J Epidemiol* 145: 10–17.

Dolk H., Shaddick G., Walls P., Grundy C. and Elliott P. (1997) *Am J Epidemiol* 145: 1–9.

Duhme H., *et al.* (1996) *Epidemiology* 7: 578–582.

Eames M., Ben-Shlomo Y. and Marmot M.G. (1993) *Br Med J* 307: 1097–1102.

Edwards J., Walters S. and Griffiths R.K. (1994) *Arch Environ Health* 49: 223–227.

Elliott P., *et al.* (1992) *J Epidemiol Commun Health* 46: 345–349.

Elliott P., *et al.* (1992) *Lancet* 339: 854–858.

Elliott P., *et al.* (1996) *Br J Cancer* 73: 702–710.

Goldberg M.S., *et al.* (1999) *Arch Environ Health* 54: 291–296.

Hodgson S., *et al.* (in press) *Am J Epidemiol*.

Kanarek M.S. (1980) *Am J Epidemiol* 112: 54–72.

Livingstone A.E., Shaddick G., Grundy C. and Elliott P. (1996) *Br Med J* 312: 676–677.

McCarron P., *et al.* (2000) *Br Med J* 320: 11–15.

Mollié A. (2000) In *Spatial Epidemiology: Methods and Applications,* eds. Elliott P., Wakefield J., Best N. and Briggs D. Oxford University Press, Oxford, pp. 267–285.

Olsen S.F., Martuzzi M. and Elliott P. (1996) *Br Med J* **313**: 863–866.

Rothenberg R.B. and Thacker S.B. (1992) In *Geographical and Environmental Epidemiology: Methods for Small-Area Studies,* eds. Elliott P., Cuzick J., English D. and Stern R. Oxford University Press, Oxford, pp. 264–277.

Simpson S., Tye R. and Diamond I. What was the real population of local areas in mid-1991? *Estimating with Confidence Project Working Paper 10,* 1995.

Staines A., and Jarup J. (2000) In *Spatial Epidemiology: Methods and Applications,* eds. Elliott P., Wakefield J., Best N. and Briggs D. Oxford University Press, Oxford, pp. 15–29.

Wilkinson P., *et al.* (1999) *Thorax* **54**: 1070–1074.

CHAPTER 4

CHARACTERISATION OF AIRBORNE PARTICULATE MATTER AND RELATED MECHANISMS OF TOXICITY: AN EXPERIMENTAL APPROACH

Kelly Bérubé, Dominique Balharry, Timothy Jones, Teresa Moreno, Patrick Hayden, Keith Sexton, Martina Hicks, Luciano Merolla, Cynthia Timblin, Arti Shukla and Brooke Mossman

1. Introduction

Atmospheric particulate matter (PM), consisting of solid and liquid particles, has both natural and anthropogenic origins. Particles are either emitted directly into the atmosphere (primary particles) or formed via chemical reactions among mixed gas phase materials and sunlight in the atmosphere (secondary particles). Typically, the major sources of primary particles are road traffic, coal combustion, industrial emissions, windblown dust and salt from sea spray. Secondary particles are mostly sulphate and nitrate salts formed by the oxidation of sulphur dioxide (SO_2) and nitrogen oxides (NO_x), and can also include gypsum formed by the reaction of ammonium sulphate with mineral particles in the atmosphere. Ambient PM may span up to six orders of magnitude in size and exhibit a wide range of physical and chemical properties. Airborne particles do not exist as

69

single components, but form complexes (aggregates) of many particle types to yield heterogeneous mixtures (Fig. 1). The composition of the particle mixtures depends on factors including location, weather conditions, season, source and emissions.

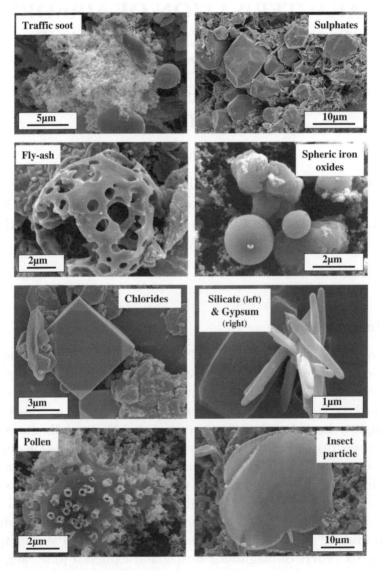

Fig. 1.   FESEM montage of the typical particle species observed in UK PM$_{10}$ samples.

The term PM_{10} (see abbreviations) is sometimes used to describe that part of the aerosol that reaches and deposits, with varying efficiency depending on individual particle size, in the thoracic airways. PM_{10} is divided into three size fractions, coarse (2.5–10 μm), fine (0.1–2.5 μm) and ultrafine (< 0.1 μm). The coarse fraction is composed of primarily crustal material such as oxides or salts of elements found in dirt, i.e. Fe, Ca, Si, Al. The major chemical components of fine particles include sulphates, nitrates, ammonium and carbonaceous material (soot particles from combustion processes). The principal source of ultrafine particles is combustion processes. The coarse fraction deposits mainly in the conducting airways, while the smaller fractions deposit further along the airways, with ultrafine particles depositing largely in the alveolar region.

1.1. *Mechanisms of Inhaled Particle Toxicity*

The current challenge facing respiratory toxicologists is to define the mechanisms by which small masses of ultrafine (Oberdorster *et al.*, 2005) or fine (Schwartz and Neas, 2000) particles can affect health. The mechanisms of toxicity are difficult to address due to the complex compositions of ambient particles. The relative contributions of particle mass, size, chemical composition or some combination of these factors, as inducers of the observed health effects, are unknown. However, it is likely that the site of particle deposition and the subsequent fate of the inhaled particles in the respiratory system are important factors (DEFRA, 2003). There is also much information which suggests that transition metals and organic compounds on the particle surfaces, along with related morphological properties such as size, shape, and aggregation, controls particle toxicity. It is believed that the inclusion of trace amounts of reactive, bioavailable (soluble) metals in the surface layers of particles increases their pathogenicity by promoting production of reactive oxygen species (ROS) at liquid-particle interfaces (Richards *et al.*, 1989; Gilmour *et al.*, 1996; Wilson *et al.*, 2002; Shukla *et al.*, 2003; Nel, 2005). Plausible mechanisms of particle action include oxidative stress, airway inflammation, oedema formation, impaired gas diffusion, cardiac dysfunction, increased plasma viscosity, immunotoxicity and neurological dysfunction (Bree and Cassee, 2000).

In this chapter, a range of complimentary particle collection, characterisation, toxicology and "omic" technologies are presented as means to explore the impact of PM within the lung (Fig. 2). Case studies are presented for each technology to show their importance in probing the mechanisms of action of particles. We have focused on the methods in use by our research group, and thus the choice of methods described in this chapter is selective.

2. Collection Methods for Airborne Particles

Historically, PM has been collected on filters with subsequent chemical analysis in the laboratory. Airborne particle collecting systems use two main methods, impaction or filtration. Collection via impaction has involved the use of a modified ChemVol Model 2400 High Volume Cascade Impactor (Thermo, UK; Moreno *et al.*, 2003; Jones *et al.*, 2005), while collection by the filtration method has utilized a horizontal elutriator system (PM$_{10}$ selective inlet head; BéruBé *et al.*, 2003a).

2.1. *Impaction Collection*

The ChemVol High Volume Cascade Impactor was originally developed at Harvard University (Kavouras *et al.*, 2000). The system requires an air flow of 800 litres/min and this requires a powerful pump. Development at Cardiff University (Moreno *et al.*, 2003; Jones *et al.*, 2005) has produced an efficient and quiet pumping system which enables the collector to be run off the UK domestic mains supplies (13AMP, 240 V). The system consists of multi-stage round-slit nozzle cascade impactors, with polyurethane foam (PUF) as the collection substrate (Kavouras and Koutrakis, 2001). The collector can be configured to collect 10–2.5 μm and 2.5–0.1 μm particles by impaction, and < 0.1 μm particles by HEPA filtration. Particles larger than 10 μm diameter are removed by a top stage fitted with a wide slit nozzle.

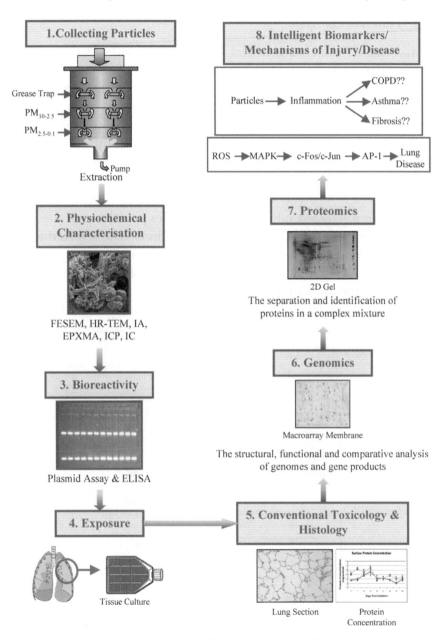

Fig. 2. Flowchart depicting the holistic approach to elucidating PM interactions within the lung environment.

2.2. *Filtration Collection*

PM$_{10}$ selective inlet heads collect airborne particles by filtration. The pumps that suck the air through the collection heads can be either powered off domestic mains 240 V or 12 V battery supplies. A flow-meter is placed in line with the pump and inlet head in order to maintain specific flow-rates. The head can be operated at 5 litres/minute to collect PM$_{2.5}$ or 30 litres/minute to collect PM$_{10}$ (BéruBé *et al.*, 1999; BéruBé *et al.*, 2003a). The system consists of a horizontal elutriator, which is also known as a classifier (Fig. 3). The horizontal elutriator separates out from an air stream all particles having a mean diameter larger than a selected value. Smaller particles pass through the classifier where they are collected on suitable filters. The selected value is referred to as the cut-off size, and theoretically no particles larger than this value will pass through the classifier. In order to achieve separation, the air is drawn through a tunnel comprising a series of horizontal plates, forcing the air into a laminar or layered flow. As air passes through the layers, particles gradually fall towards the lower plate, with the larger particles falling faster.

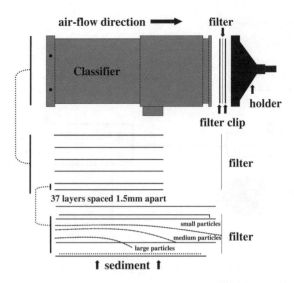

Fig. 3.   A schematic diagramme of a horizontal elutriator, (classifier), denoting the process of particle filtration.

2.3. *Filter Selection*

The choice of filter is the most important aspect of sampling, especially if compositional analysis or microscopical investigation of the collected particles is required. In the latter case, membrane filters are the most suitable. For compositional analysis, polycarbonate filters are ideal since they dissolve easily in organic solvents with minimal trace element. This enables the collected material to be recovered within a small volume of solvent for chemical analysis. Polycarbonate filters are excellent substrates for analysis by scanning electron microscopy due to their smooth surfaces. Moreover, particles can be easily washed from the filters for further processing, e.g. X-ray microanalysis. Their optical transparency properties also make it possible to observe PM *in situ* on filters, hence reducing contamination (BéruBé *et al.*, 2003b). Finally, some polycarbonate filters are non-hygroscopic, have a low, reproducible tare weight, and do not need to be pre- and post-conditioned at 50% relative humidity and constant temperature for gravimetric analysis.

Polyurethane foam is recommended as a substrate for the ChemVol High Volume Cascade Impactor (Thermo, UK). It is textured and the porous surface results in negligible particle "bounce-off" and "re-entrainment" losses. The particle size "cut-off" is controlled by the air flow rate, where the width and the height of the slit are above the substrate. The very high air impaction speeds mean that the foam does not just act as a textured surface to entrap particles, but air is also forced sideways through the wall of the trench in the foam created by the air flow and particles are effectively "filtered" out. The foam therefore acts as a hybrid substrate/filter.

3. Analysis Methods for Airborne Particles

3.1. *Electron Microscopy and Image Analysis*

The examination of the size, shape and surface characteristics of particles requires the use of *in situ* high resolution transmission and field emission scanning electron microscopy (HR-TEM, FESEM; BéruBé *et al.*, 2003b; Jones *et al.*, 2005). TEM provides information about the

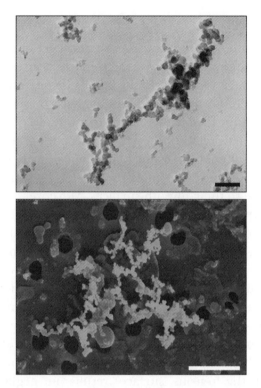

Fig. 4. The ultrastructural properties of DEP particles as observed by TEM (*top image*) and by SEM (*bottom image*).

ultrastructural properties of particles by passing a beam of electrons through them, whereas SEM scans the surface of the particles with an electron beam to produce an image of the particle surface (Fig. 4). Quantitative data of particle morphology can be obtained by image analysis (BéruBé *et al.*, 2003a). EM images are first digitally captured, processed and measurements of primary feature data, i.e. shape and size, made automatically using standard IA software. IA is suitable for the determination of morphological parameters including equivalent spherical diameter (ESD), which in turn can be used to derive mass, volume and surface area data of particulate matter samples (Fig. 5; BéruBé *et al.*, 1999). ESD can be related to aerodynamic diameter and thus to metrics such as PM_{10}.

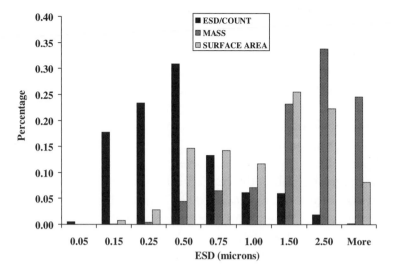

Fig. 5. Particle size distribution of a DEP sample determined by measuring the ESD of particle aggregates from TEM micrographs (BéruBé *et al.*, 1999).

3.2. *Elemental Analysis*

The elemental composition of PM can be characterised using a variety of methods, e.g. inductively coupled plasma–mass spectrometry (ICP-MS) and ion chromatography (IC). The most convenient method is electron probe X-ray microanalysis (EPXMA) in conjunction with EM (BéruBé *et al.*, 2003b; Jones *et al.*, 2005). This non-destructive technique, where samples may be reused for other analysis (e.g. mass spectrometry), is ideal for analysis of microquantities of materials and no previous sample treatment is required. Although a range of inorganic elements can be detected (e.g. Ca^{2+}, Cl^-), no indication of the amount of actual compounds (e.g. $CaCl_2$) can be obtained in the sample. EPXMA involves particles being viewed at high magnification in a TEM or SEM that is fitted with an energy dispersive X-ray detector. A fine beam of electrons emitted from the TEM is directed at the particles, causing them to emit X-rays of characteristic energies depending on the elements present. Importantly, EPXMA permits the correlation of structural information with chemical content. These correlations are particularly evident when using a qualitative X-ray mapping technique known as "speed-mapping". This method can be used to determine the relative spatial distribution of elements in a structurally heterogeneous sampling field of particulate matter (Fig. 6; BéruBé *et al.*, 2003b). The elemental organic carbon compounds (EOCC), most likely in the form of DEP, are on average 30 nm in diameter with an estimated volume of $1 \times 10^{-5} \, \mu m^3$ (BéruBé *et al.*, 1999).

Inductively coupled plasma-mass spectrometry (ICP-MS) is a very sensitive technique that can detect elements at concentrations of 0.1 parts per trillion (ppt), and it is one of the most powerful methods for the determination of the concentrations of trace elements in environmental samples (Yang *et al.*, 2002). Sample throughput using the technique is high. When analysing whole particulate samples, i.e. both soluble and insoluble components (Moreno *et al.*, 2003, 2004; see below), solid sampling is possible, but this technique usually involves matrix-matching problems between standards and samples, and is less sensitive than the analysis of solutions. Therefore, it is desirable to dissolve the samples and analyse the dilute solution.

Hotplate nitric acid digestion does not reach high enough temperatures to dissolve much of the constituent material of carbonaceous rich particulate samples. Conventional bomb digestion operates at higher temperatures, but the process is slow (16–18 hours) due to the long warm up and cool down times required (Neas and Collins, 1988). Microwave dissolution at elevated pressures allows reagents to reach higher temperatures than the hotplate method, and thus has the advantage of more effective and rapid sample dissolution. As sample preparation times are short and vessels are closed during the microwave procedure, contamination from environmental exposure is minimised, therefore analytical blanks are improved and volatile loss is prevented (Neas and Collins, 1988). Analysis of the soluble fraction from particulate samples is much more straightforward, requiring only the soluble material to be extracted into deionised water.

3.3. *In Vitro and In Vivo Characterisation*

Physicochemical characterisation of PM samples can produce a great deal of information regarding their potential toxicity. These results

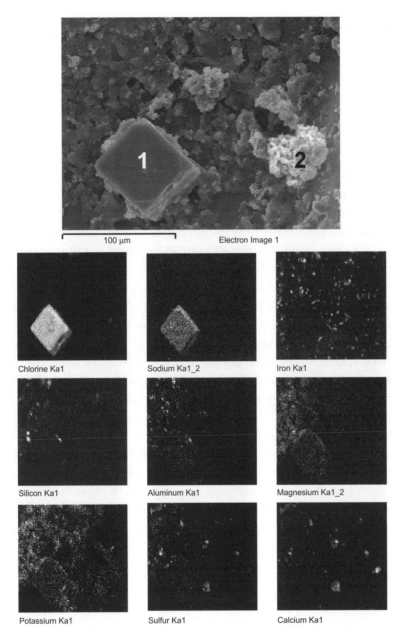

Fig. 6. Example of the multi-element capability of SEM-EPXMA: (*top*) electron micrograph of particles (1 = salt crystal; 2 = soot particles) suspended onto a PUF coated with palladium/gold and mounted onto an aluminium SEM stub. (*bottom*) corresponding digital X-ray map revealing the chemical heterogeneity of the PM10 particles.

should be compared with the bioreactivity of the samples to identify potential factors that may be associated with the observed health
effects of ambient particles. Studies of bioreactivity range from *in vitro*
assays to more complex *in vivo* studies.

3.4. *Plasmid Assay*

The plasmid assay is a simple *in vitro* assay which detects the presence of reactive oxygen species (ROS) at the surface of particulate
samples. The technique requires only a small sample of PM (soluble
and non-soluble fractions; 500–1,000 μg) and is an ideal means for
an initial examination of the bioreactivity of PM, without the need
to sacrifice the large amount of sample required for *in vivo* studies.
The basis of the plasmid assay is the quantification of the damage to
a plasmid caused by incubation with varying concentrations of the
particulate sample of interest. The plasmid φX174 RF is used, since
it was found to be of the optimum size to be receptive to damage at
suitably low PM concentrations. The damage to the plasmid occurs
in three stages; firstly, the plasmid DNA is converted from the tight
supercoiled (undamaged) form into the relaxed (damaged) form.
Once sufficient damage has occurred, the plasmid ring breaks, leading to the linear form. The final stage is the complete fragmentation
of the DNA. These different forms of the plasmid have different elec-
trophoretic mobilities and can be separated using gel electrophoresis.
The gel is examined under UV light and the intensity of each band,
and therefore the % DNA damage is quantified. A regression line can
be plotted to allow calculation of the amount of the sample necessary
to cause 50% damage (TD_{50}) to the supercoiled DNA (above that
observed with the water plus plasmid alone control).

3.5. *In Vivo Techniques*

Intratracheal instillation

Intratracheal instillation is frequently used in the studies of the toxicity of both soluble and insoluble particulate matter. The technique
allows the instantaneous delivery of a PM dose, in a small volume of

carrier liquid, directly into the lung. This avoids any deposition in the upper respiratory tract (Osier and Oberdorster, 1997). However, instillation is obviously not a physiological route for human exposure and differences in particle distribution, clearance and pattern of injury have been found, when compared with inhalation studies (Osier and Oberdorster, 1997). Some argue that deposition in the nasopharyngeal region of the respiratory tract is an important factor, and instillation of a relatively large dose into the lung can also cause an inflammatory response that would not occur, if the particles accumulated gradually (Henderson *et al.*, 1995). It is also argued that the carrier liquid may have an effect (Henderson *et al.*, 1995). This can be investigated with the use of appropriate controls. Once the particulate dose has been administered, effects on the experimental animal after a suitable time period can be investigated and compared with those found in control animals. Lung damage can be determined by investigating changes in lung/body weight ratio, in acellular lavage protein to monitor epithelial permeability, and in changes of free cell counts to assess the extent of airway/alveolar inflammation (Murphy *et al.*, 1998).

3.6. *Case Study: Characterisation of PM in Port Talbot, South Wales*

Port Talbot is a coastal town with 135,000 inhabitants in South Wales, UK. The town is bounded to the north by a motorway and is heavily industrialised with a steelwork factory located immediately south and southeast of the town. Airborne samples were collected to investigate the relationship between source apportionment and wind direction. The collector was located behind Groeswen Hospital that lies just 100 meters southwest of the extremely busy London to South Wales motorway, 100 meters north of an urban access road, 800 meters northeast of the steel producing factory, and around 2,500 meters from the sea (Moreno *et al.*, 2004). The traffic flow in the immediately surrounding area is estimated to be 50,000 to 55,000 vehicles per day (DETR, 2002). Samples are described for four periods of varying wind direction.

A total of 69.11 mg of $PM_{10-2.5}$ and 127.06 mg of $PM_{2.5}$ was collected over four sampling periods in a total of 15 days. The masses of particles collected varied with the wind direction:

- SW/SE: mixed steelworks and motorway sources — 0.90 mg/hr
- SE (motorway) and NW (Port Talbot town): 0.68 mg/hr
- NE: 0.32 mg/hr

The $PM_{2.5}/PM_{10-2.5}$ ratios also varied:

- SW/SE : 1.12
- NW   : 1.76
- NE   : 2.63
- SE   : 2.67

Total PM_{10} air pollution levels over the same periods were available from the UK Department of Environment, Food and Rural Affairs (DEFRA) monitoring site in Port Talbot, located 50 m SE from the high-volume collector (DEFRA, http://www.stanger.co.uk). These data revealed stable pollution levels (mostly 10–20 $\mu g/m^3$) for the NW and SE samples, and generally lower levels (mostly 5–15 $\mu g/m^3$) for the NE sample. With the exception of the mixed SW/SE sample, the only time when pollution levels exceeded 30 $\mu g/m^3$ was during the Friday morning peak traffic period on 19 October, when the NE sample was being collected. The SW/SE sample again showed background levels of 10–20 $\mu g/m^3$, but included two prominent pollution episodes. The first of these occurred in the afternoon of the 29 October when levels exceeded 25 $\mu g/m^3$ for 10 hours and reached a peak of 62 $\mu g/m^3$. During this time, winds were blowing from the WSW (230–260°) and the collecting site lay directly downwind of the main steelworks furnaces. This pollution episode coincided with the period of highest rainfall measured during the collecting time. The second pollution episode, although recording a dramatic 94 $\mu g/m^3$, was transient (one reading), occurred when the wind was in the SE (100°), and its origin was unclear. Finally, comparing the DEFRA data with rainfall recorded by the Met Office, during the collection of the NE and the SW/SE samples, exposed no obvious link between mass recorded and the amount of precipitation was found. The variations in particulate ($\mu g/m^3$) appear to be primarily linked to traffic (in the SE and NE samples), factory and traffic emissions (in the SW/SE sample). The NW sample shows only minor (probably traffic-related) variations, with mass collected decreasing with more northerly directed winds (i.e. away from the town).

3.7. *SEM Characterisation*

Four samples (NE, NW, SE and mixed SW/SE) were obtained as part of the collecting period under different wind directions. The estimated relative percentages of the different types of particles in the samples as total PM_{10} (coarse and fine fractions together) are shown in Fig. 7. Elemental organic carbon compounds (EOCC) and nitrates were the most abundant particles in all four samples, in both the coarse and fine fractions. Sulphate particles were mostly attributed to calcium sulphate (gypsum) in the coarser $PM_{10-2.5}$ fraction, and ammonium sulphate in the $PM_{2.5}$ fraction. This has been observed elsewhere (Querol *et al.*, 2001; Ho *et al.*, 2003; Moreno *et al.*, 2003), and seems to be true of all four samples in this study. The chloride particles found in the four samples were present only in the coarse fraction

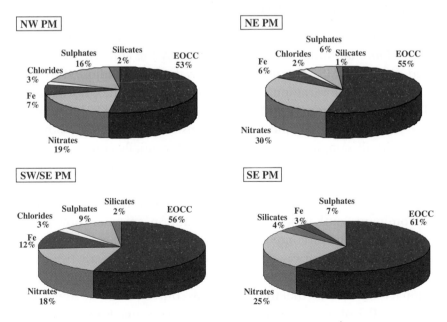

Fig. 7. Port Talbot PM elemental composition derived from SEM-EPXMA.

and were absent from the SE sample. Silicate particles were concentrated in the coarser fraction of all four samples, and the relative rates at which they were collected can be compared by calculating the number of silicate $PM_{10-2.5}$ present in 500 SEM analyses divided by the number collection hours (SH500). Thus, the samples with the highest amount of silicate (and therefore the highest SH500) are those from the SE (SH500 = 0.8) and NW (SH500 = 0.7), both of which were collected under dry conditions. Lower values are found in the mixed SW/SE (SH500 = 0.3) and NE (SH500 = 0.1) samples. The silicates analysed were preferentially Al-Si-rich (felsic silicates; Moreno *et al.*, 2004), including quartz, feldspar and mainly clay minerals. Finally, relative to other samples, Fe-rich particles were most numerous in the mixed SW/SE sample, followed in turn by the NE, NW and SE samples. Fe-rich particle numbers were more abundant in the coarse fraction in the samples derived from the NE, SE and NW, whereas the mixed sample containing SW-derived material shows similar amounts for both fractions, indicating an increase in Fe in the $PM_{2.5}$.

3.8. *ICP-MS Characterisation*

Metal contents of the four samples collected in Port Talbot, according to dominant wind directions: NE, SE, SW/SE and NW, were analysed using ICP-MS. The mass concentrations were adjusted to take into account the variations in collection rate (mg/hr), normalising all parts per million (ppm) values to those of the SW/SE sample (the heaviest one). Fe and Zn were consistently the most abundant metals in all samples, with Zn being preferentially concentrated in the soluble fraction. The data, however, revealed marked differences depending on the dominant wind direction. The SW/SE sample, partly derived from the direction of the steelworks, and including a prominent south-westerly-derived pollution episode, showed the highest overall metal content, with amounts of total metals nearly double that of the motorway-only derived sample, and nearly five times that of the town. This increase in metal content was even more striking when it is considered that this sample was sourced from the steelworks for only 30% of the collection time. The excess metals in this sample were Fe, Mn, Ni and Zn ($\Sigma = 40{,}730$ ppm). Compared with the SE motorway sample, the sample containing steelworks-derived metals suggested a drop in the traffic-related metals Pb, V Ti, As, and Ce. In contrast, the sample containing the lowest metal content was that which was sourced across Port Talbot town, a direction avoiding both motorway and steelworks. This was illustrated by the fact that the total burden of Fe, Zn, Mn and Ni ($\Sigma = 8,107$ ppm) in this "town" sample was $< 20\%$ of that which was measured in the mixed SW/SE (steelworks/motorway) sample.

The sample collected when winds were sourced from the SE, along the motorway corridor, exhibited considerable amounts of metal content (Fe, Zn, Mn and Ni $\Sigma = 20,735$ ppm). This sample had the highest levels of Pb, V, Cu, Ti, As and Ce. The elevated level of Pb (2,044 ppm) was especially noticeable. The sample collected when winds were blowing from the NE quadrant across the adjacent motorway at a high angle, also demonstrated enhanced levels of Pb (1,856 ppm), and similar amounts of Fe, Zn, Mn and Ni ($\Sigma = 18,018$ ppm). The dramatic difference in metal content between the NW and SE samples emphasised the important contribution that road traffic makes to the atmospheric metal aerosol burden, but may also reflect re-suspension of particles originally derived from the steelworks. Metals appearing significantly in the soluble fraction included Zn, As, and Cu, whereas Ni, Ti and Mo were similar to Fe in being relatively less soluble. Another potential factor influencing the behaviour and transport of metals in the atmosphere was aerosol size. In this experiment, both Zn and Pb were always found preferentially concentrated in the finer ($PM_{2.5}$) fraction.

3.9. *Case Study: In Vitro Effects of Water-soluble Metals Found in Particles Collected in London in 1958*

Inductively coupled plasma mass spectrometry (BéruBé *et al.*, 2003b), of a black smoke (BS) sample collected in London in 1958 (Whittaker, 2003; Whittaker *et al.*, 2004), was performed in order to discover which metals were present in the water-soluble fraction of the PM and their concentrations (Merolla and Richards, 2005); BéruBé *et al.*, 2005). A surrogate preparation of the bioavailable metals present was then generated. The TD_{50} value of the surrogate metal mixture in the plasmid assay was $0.44\,\mu g\ ml^{-1}$. The soluble material from the London sample gave a TD_{50} value of $162.5\,\mu g\,ml^{-1}$ (Whittaker et al., 2004) and this contained $0.55\,\mu g\,ml^{-1}$ of metal. Therefore, the bioavailable metal content of the 1958 London sample accounted for a TD_{50} value of $0.55\,\mu g\ ml^{-1}$ in the scission assay (Merolla and Richards, 2005).

The bioreactivity of each metal species was determined via the plasmid assay. The most bioreactive metals were found to be Fe^{2+}, Cu^{2+}, Fe^{3+}, V^{4+}, whereas Zn^{2+}, Pb^{2+}, As^{3+}, V^{5+}, and Mn^{2+} had very low bioreactivity. The oxidative impact of combinations of metals was also investigated, focusing on the redox inactive metal Zn^{2+} and four of the more bio-reactive metals, Cu^{2+}, Fe^{3+}, V^{4+}, Fe^{2+}. Dose-dependent synergy between zinc and Fe^{3+}, zinc and $V^{4+}$and zinc and Cu^{2+} was found. Little evidence of synergistic effects was found for zinc and Fe^{2+}. The analysis of the metals in differing oxidation states revealed that valency played an essential role in oxidative capacity. Fe^{2+} was more than 15 times more damaging than Fe^{3+}. In addition, V^{4+} was highly bio-reactive in comparison with V^{5+}. It was possible creating a bioreactivity hierarchy of these metals where $Fe^{2+} > Cu^{2+} > Fe^{3+} > V^{4+} > Zn^{2+} > As^{3+} = Pb^{2+} = Mn^{2+} = V^{5+}$.

The ability of Fe^{2+} to exert the greatest oxidative threat is consistent with existing research, which has shown that Fe^{2+} has a significant ability in generating ROS (including hydroxyl radicals via Fenton-type reactions [Urbanski and Beresewicz, 2000]). Evidence has also been presented to show that Cu^{2+} poses a redox threat to DNA (Stohs and Bagchi 1995). Zn^{2+} presents no redox threat toward DNA, due to its existence in only one oxidation state. However, Zn^{2+} is able to hydrolyse ester bonds, which may explain the observed synergistic effect between it and other metals. The oxidation state of the metal used with zinc seems to be an important factor and it seems more probable that the zinc is having an effect on the metal ion itself, as opposed to the plasmid. The data supports previous in vitro findings with cellular systems, which have shown that exposure to zinc and copper mixture resulted in significantly greater epithelial toxicity responses than did exposure to zinc or copper alone (Pagan et al., 2003). Therefore, evidence was found for the role of water-soluble, redox-active, transition metals in the oxidative bioreactivity of the most abundant metals found in a typical historical London sample. It appears that low valence transition metals may be a key to determining particulate matter-induce oxidation.

4. *In Vitro* Human Airway Epithelial Models

The study of the respiratory effects of environmental pollutants requires the availability of appropriate experimental models. Animal models including rodent, canine and primate species have traditionally been used for inhalation toxicology studies. However, animal models suffer from a variety of limitations. For example, significant differences between human and animal respiratory physiology make dosimetry and particle disposition results obtained from animal models difficult to extrapolate to humans (Schlesinger, 1985). Significant differences in xenobiotic metabolizing enzymes also exist between animal models and humans. Therefore, metabolism-dependent toxicity, carcinogenicity and xenobiotic clearance data derived from animal models are also difficult to extrapolate to humans (Buckpitt *et al.*, 2002; Green, 2000; Cruzan, 2002). Furthermore, animal models are becoming increasingly impractical for modern high throughput screening applications, where large numbers of test articles or limited quantities of test articles need to be studied. Ethical considerations of animal use in toxicology experiments are also a serious concern (Flecknell, 2002). Reliable *in vitro* human models for inhalation toxicology studies are thus desirable.

Normal human nasal, tracheal/bronchial and alveolar epithelial cells can be cultured *in vitro* and have been routinely utilized in toxicology and basic research for a number of years. However, submerged monolayer cultures of undifferentiated epithelial cells grown on plastic substrates do not adequately model the physiologic and biochemical properties of differentiated epithelial tissues. For example, undifferentiated submerged monolayer cultures do not develop cilia, secrete mucins or develop the tight junctional complexes necessary for the formation of tight epithelial barriers. Additionally, growth in submerged culture on nonporous plastic substrates does not allow for appropriate permeation studies or application of formulations which may include particles, powders or other water insoluble materials.

4.1. The EpiAirway™ In Vitro Human Tracheal/Bronchial Epithelial Model

For many research laboratories interested in utilizing highly differentiated air-liquid interface (ALI) airway culture systems, it is convenient and economical to obtain fully developed differentiated ALI cultures in a ready-to-use state from commercial sources. One such model system is the EpiAirway™ *in vitro* human airway epithelial model (MatTek Corp., Ashland, MA). This system is produced from normal human tracheal/bronchial epithelial cells cultured on a variety of individual and high throughput screening culture inserts formats. The cultures display the highly differentiated pseudostratified, mucociliary morphology typical of *in vivo* tracheal/bronchial epithelium. LMs of a typical EpiAirway culture section is shown in Fig. 8(a). Corresponding TEM images reveals additional details of ciliated cells and tight junctional complexes [Fig. 8(c)]. Normal airway epithelium is shown in Fig. 8(b).

Barrier properties of EpiAirway cultures can be evaluated by measurement of transepithelial electrical resistance (TEER). *In vivo* TEER values are difficult to measure. However, values of about 100--300 $\Omega \times cm^2$ have been reported for excised tracheal epithelia of various species, including humans (Knowles *et al.*, 1984; Ballad and Taylor, 1994; Joris and Quinton, 1991). EpiAirway cultures typically develop TEER in the range of 300–500 $\Omega \times cm^2$.

The objective of this case study was to characterise a model of toxicity in human respiratory epithelia, following exposure to nicotine, a particle phase component of tobacco smoke (TSC). EpiAirway cultures were equilibrated overnight in fresh media. Nicotine was solubilised in phosphate buffered saline (PBS) to a range of concentrations, and 100 μl was applied to the apical surface of each culture. This was incubated for 24 hours in a 37°C, 5% CO_2 incubator. Following exposure to nicotine, the apical surface was washed with 300 μl PBS. The PBS wash was retained for protein analysis (Bradford, 1976), to identify altered levels of mucin in response to nicotine. Colorimetric assay generated data on the total amount of protein contained within the apical surface wash (Fig. 20; *top*). The tissue cultures were then transferred into fresh media, and the used media kept for cytokine

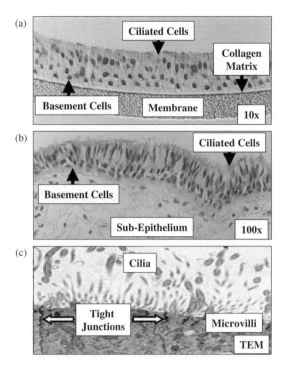

Fig. 8. Light and TEM micrographs (MG) of an EpiAirway culture. (a) EpiAirway culture. (b) Normal human airway epithelium. (c) TEM EpiAirway culture showing cilia, microvilli and tight junctional complexes.

analysis. Having been in contact with the basal surface of the tissue, cytokine secretions should have permeated directly into the media. Cytokine measurements were carried out using Proteoplex™ Protein Arrays (Merck Biosciences, Nottingham, UK), which contain 12 different human cytokines. Finally, TEER and MTT measurements were taken (as described previously) to determine the tissue integrity and cell viability. On completion of the toxicological analysis, the tissue was stored in RNAlater (Qiagen, West Sussex, UK) to prevent RNA degradation over time. When the samples were ready for use, the tissue was separated from the collagen matrix on which it rests. At this point, QIAzol lysis reagent (Qiagen, West Sussex, UK) was simultaneously used to isolate RNA for genomic studies, and protein for proteomic analysis. Nicotine was found to produce a dose-dependent increase in the total protein content of the apical surface wash fluid. There seemed to be a threshold of effect at a 50 mM concentration of nicotine, where the protein content of the wash fluid rose rapidly at higher concentrations. The MTT and TEER assays also showed clear effects with high (125 mM) concentrations, producing approximately 50% reduction in MTT and the abolition of epithelial electrical resistance.

5. Toxicogenomics and Gene Expression Studies

Genomics as a technique may be defined in terms of the structural, functional and comparative analysis of genomes and gene products from a wide variety of organisms. The characterisation of the genetic responses of cells and tissues to a variety of toxicant and chemical insults is known as toxicogenomics. An important step in the pursuit of this is in defining gene expression profiles. This compares patterns of expression in different tissues and at different developmental stages, in normal and diseased states, or when under defined *in vitro* conditions.

The current approach for simultaneously analysing multiple genes is the hybridisation of the entire complementary DNA (cDNA) populations to nucleic acid arrays. Macroarrays are most commonly used to measure the levels of expression (mRNA abundance) of thousands of genes simultaneously. For the majority of genes, changes in mRNA abundance are related to changes in protein concentration (Lockhart and Winzeler, 2000), protein synthesis being dependent on mRNA expression. The transcription of genomic DNA (gDNA) to produce mRNA is the first step in protein synthesis. Therefore, the expression profile of a collection of genes is a major determinant of cellular phenotype and function. Differences in gene expression are indicative of both morphological and phenotypic differences, as well as of cellular responses to environmental stimuli. In terms of understanding the function of genes, knowing when, where, and to what extent a gene is expressed, is key to understanding the activity and biological roles of its encoded protein. In addition, changes in the expression patterns can provide information about regulatory mechanisms and broader cellular functions and biochemical pathways (Cox *et al.*, 2005).

The construction of an array is based on immobilising DNA sequences at specific locations on a solid support. The sequences were originally generated by PCR from a plasmid library, and range approximately from 250 bp to 2 Kbp. The gene array method exploits the specificity and affinity of complementary base pairing between labelled experimental cDNA and the immobilised DNA sequences. A cDNA copy of an RNA probe is generated by reverse transcription (RT) of total RNA or purified polyA mRNA extracted from tissue. During the RT reaction, cDNA is either directly labelled with fluorescent or radioisotope tags, or reactive side groups for subsequent labelling (e.g. Biotin). The cDNA is then hybridised to the immobilised DNA sequences on the array.

The extent of differential hybridisation to each individual sequence on the array can be determined by fluorescence, phosphorimager analysis or similar techniques. Following quantification, the relative abundance of each of the gene sequences in two or more biological samples can be compared (Brown and Botstein, 1999). Arrays can contain sequences selected to investigate specific endpoints or pathways, or they can include genes representing a wide range of biological processes. A number of "housekeeping genes" are included to aid in the normalisation of data. The expression of housekeeping genes is expected to be stable under a wide range of conditions.

5.1. *Case Study: Bioreactivity of Metals in UK Particulate Matter*

The water-soluble fraction of PM is generally rich in bioavailable metals, especially transition metals, and has been shown to have great oxidative capacity (Greenwell *et al.*, 2002; Whittaker *et al.*, 2004; Merolla and Richards, 2005). It has been suggested that the adverse health effects associated with PM, predominantly pulmonary and cardiac disorders, are linked to the metal content of the samples. Despite the volume of literature on this topic, the mechanisms of action of bioreactive metals are poorly understood. The application of genomic technology permits investigations of the genetic mechanisms underlying the toxicity of bioreactive metals, and has the potential to identify candidate genes responsible for eliciting these disease mechanisms.

The primary objective of this case study was to profile differential gene expression at the transcriptional level within the lungs, caused by the instillation of a metal mixture (MM). The mixture contained three times the concentration of metals found in London PM (Cu^{2+}, V^{2+}, Fe^{2+} and Zn^{2+}, e.g. Merolla and Richards, 2005). Rats were exposed to this mixture. Details of the methods used may be found in Balharry (2005). Control rats were exposed to an equivalent volume of saline. Four hours after dosing, the lungs were excised and snap frozen in liquid nitrogen, after which the right apical lobe was homogenized and phenol-chloroform extraction was used to isolate total RNA. The purity and quantity of the RNA was confirmed using spectrophotometry and gel electrophoresis.

A nylon platform macroarray was used to explore the changes in mRNA expression between MM dosed and control lungs. The arrays comprised 207 cDNAs, doubly spotted onto a positively charged membrane, including plasmid and bacteriophage DNA as negative controls (confirmation of hybridisation specificity), as well as housekeeping genes (positive controls). The experimental RNA samples were reverse transcribed to incorporate ^{32}P, and the resulting labelled cDNA probes were then hybridised onto the membrane overnight. Finally, the membranes were exposed to a phosphorimager screen which was scanned. The resulting image was quantified using AtlasImage 2.0 (Clontech™) computer software. A quantitative measure of gene expression was calculated by subtracting the background intensity from the spot intensities (Balharry, 2005).

Processing of the arrays ($n = 3$), followed by quantitative comparative analysis, gave rise to 35 genes with fold changes greater than 1.5 (15 up-regulated and 20 down-regulated in MM treated lung). Of the 35 genes selected, 19 were omitted due to CV values falling outside the range of 0–0.3. Finally, a t-test was used to gauge whether the difference between control and MM treated genes was significant. The results obtained from the t-test indicated that 13 of the genes were significantly altered. Ten of the genes were significantly down-regulated and 3 genes were significantly up-regulated. These genes fell primarily into three biologically related families (e.g. metabolism, cell cycle and stress response), that accounted for a total of 68% of all the genes altered. The statistically significantly altered genes are listed in Table 1.

The results obtained from this study support evidence that transition metals found in PM contribute to oxidative stress within the lung (Merolla and Richards, 2005). The evidence suggests that the control of antioxidants such a glutathione is involved in a pivotal role in combating this type of damage. Overall, the toxicogenomic analysis supports the data found in previous studies, which indicated that the water-soluble metals have a redox effect on the lung. The primary genomic responses revolved around up-regulating redox-specific stress mechanisms and metabolism pathways in order to neutralise the xenobiotics.

6. Molecular Bioreactivity of Different Particles *In Vitro*

The physico-chemical properties of PM may dictate their bioreactivity in the cells of the respiratory tract, as well as their capacity to cause or promote respiratory disease. The documented effects of PM on pulmonary epithelial cells, specifically the cell signalling pathways that appear to play a role in proliferation and apoptosis, are important in a number of lung diseases. Upon inhalation, particles impinge on the pulmonary epithelium. The epithelial cell of the lung is a cell type that is affected in asthma, chronic bronchitis, lung cancer and a variety of other respiratory diseases. In addition, the alveolar Type 2 cell may be important in chemokine production and the elaboration of cytokines that are intrinsic to inflammation, proliferation and fibrogenesis (Mossman and Churg, 1998). Moreover, uptake of PM and a number of other particles and fibres have been demonstrated in epithelial cells and human lung parenchyma (Churg, 1996; Churg and Brauer, 1997). Although alveolar macrophages accumulate at sites of particle deposition and phagocytize PM and particles *in vitro*, attention in a number of laboratories has focused on PM-induced molecular responses in SV40 T antigen-transformed human epithelial cell lines (BEAS-2B) and Type 2 cells lines derived from mice (C10) (Malkinson *et al.*, 1997) or rats (RLE) (Driscoll *et al.*, 1995).

Table 1. Significantly altered genes in MM treated lung tissue. Fold change, CV, p value and functional classification of each gene is represented.

Name	Genebank ID	Ratio	CV Saline	CV MM	P-value	Functional Group
Growth-related c-myc-responsive protein (RCL)	U82591	−1.518	0.170	0.122	0.035	Cell cycle
M-phase inducer phosphatase 2 (MPI2)	D16237	−1.568	0.134	0.255	0.041	Cell cycle
Cyclin-dependent kinase 5 (CDK5)	L02121	−1.932	0.116	0.012	0.024	Cell cycle
DNA topoisomerase IIB (TOP2B)	D14046	−1.579	0.126	0.128	0.013	DNA synthesis, recombination and repair
Extracellular signal regulated kinase1 (ERK1)	M61177	−1.538	0.116	0.145	0.015	Intracellular transducers, effectors and modulators
Heme oxygenase 1 (HMOX1; HO1)	J02722	1.952	0.245	0.079	0.005	Metabolism
Heme oxygenase 2 (HMOX2; HO2)	J05405	−1.504	0.138	0.148	0.027	Metabolism
Glutathione reductase (GSR)	U73174	1.812	0.293	0.077	0.012	Metabolism
Glutathione S-transferase Yb subunit (GSTM2)	J02592	−1.559	0.069	0.248	0.023	Metabolism
Calcium binding protein 2 (CABP2)	M86870	−1.516	0.085	0.171	0.014	Post translational modification and folding
Microsomal glutathione S-transferase (GST12)	J03752	−1.743	0.217	0.250	0.046	Stress response
Glutathione S-transferase subunit 5 theta (GST5-5)	X67654	1.643	0.217	0.080	0.012	Stress response
Eukaryotic peptide chain release factor subunit 1 (ERF1)	M75715	−1.591	0.170	0.114	0.025	Translation

As opposed to primary cell cultures, these lines yield the large numbers of cells required for most molecular and biological techniques. Confluent cells have been used since they best mimic the contiguous arrangement of the lung epithelial cells *in vivo*.

6.1. Case Studies – Exposure of Pulmonary Epithelial Cell Lines to Ambient PM

An advantage of using cell cultures is that responses can be related to the numbers of particles and/or particle surface area per cell or area of culture dish, using sophisticated cell-imaging techniques. In studies described below (Timblin *et al.*, 1998), PM_{10} samples were originally collected on glass or Teflon filters from the Burlington, Vermont (USA) monitoring station, using a Wedding collection apparatus. A $PM_{2.5}$ fraction was prepared by sonication in double-distilled water and filtration through a polycarbonate filter with a 2.5 μm (diameter) pore size. Particles were lyophilised and stored at $-80°C$ until use. In recent work, $PM_{2.5}$ has been collected on Teflon filters and treated identically. Fine and ultrafine TiO_2 and ultrafine carbon black (CB) particles have also been used in all experiments, and their physicochemical properties characterised. PM and other particles were resuspended in a balanced salt solution and added to confluent cultures in low serum (0.5%) or serum-less media at a range of concentrations. Cells exposed to particles have been assessed for cytotoxicity (Timblin *et al.*, 2002) and assayed for apoptosis (BéruBé *et al.*, 1996). These studies show that concentrations of PM or ultrafine particles at $\leq 10\,\mu g/cm^2$ (dish area) are non-cytotoxic.

6.2. Molecular Mechanisms of Toxicity

Recent evidence indicates that PM can stimulate intracellular signalling pathways leading to the activation of nuclear transcription factors, i.e. Activator Protein–1 (AP-1), Nuclear Factor-kappa B (NF-*κ*B), and changes in gene expression (Timblin *et al.*, 1998; Shukla *et al.*, 2000). Activation of these signalling cascades may be linked to the production of reactive oxygen species (ROS), catalysed by Fenton-type reactions with transition metals in particle samples, or alternatively, generated by an oxidative burst during phagocytosis of the particles by pulmonary cells (Shulka *et al.*, 2003). The phenotypic endpoints of these signalling cascades may be determined by the patterns of gene expression and may include changes in cell proliferation, survival, inflammation and cell death (apoptosis).

$PM_{2.5}$ has been shown to cause activation of the c-Jun Kinase/Stress-activated protein kinase (JNK) cascade and DNA synthesis in rat alveolar Type 2 epithelial (RLE-6TN) cell lines (Timblin *et al.*, 1998). The JNK pathway is characterised by a series of phosphorylation events initiated at the cell surface that ultimately lead to the activation of JNK and to the phosphorylation of multiple nuclear transcription factors, such as AP-1. The protooncogenes c-*jun* and c-*fos* are members of the immediate-early response gene family that encode subunits (Jun/Jun homodimers or Jun/Fos heterodimers) of the AP-1 complex that are involved in the transition of the G1 phase and entry into the S phase of the cell cycle (Angel and Karin, 1991). In pulmonary epithelial cell lines (RLE-6TN) exposed to non-cytotoxic concentrations of PM, an increase in JNK activity is associated with increases in the levels of phosphorylated c-Jun protein and the transcriptional activation of the AP-1 dependent genes (Timblin *et al.*, 1998). These changes are accompanied by increases in the numbers of cells incorporating 5'-bromodeoxyuridine, a marker of unscheduled DNA synthesis, and total cell numbers. Thus, early molecular changes lead to increased cell proliferation, a critical event in the pathogenesis of a number of respiratory disorders and diseases, but also of importance in lung repair.

6.3. *Proto-oncogenes*

The patterns of the *fos* (c-*fos*, *fra*-1, *fra*-2, *fos*B) and *jun* (c-*jun*, *jun*B, *jun*D) family gene expression are different in Type 2 epithelial cell lines (C10) exposed to low or high, cytotoxic concentrations of PM and may be directly related, respectively, to the phenotypic endpoints of cell proliferation and apoptosis observed. In cells exposed to high concentrations ($50\,\mu g/cm^2$ dish) of PM, early but transient increases in mRNA levels of all *jun* and *fos* family genes are observed. In contrast, low doses of PM stimulate striking but delayed increases in mRNA levels for *fra*-1, *fra*-2 and c-*jun* genes (Timblin *et al.*, 1998). Elevated levels of c-*fos* are not observed at any time period in cells exposed to low doses of PM. In some cell types, expression of c-*fos* is associated with apoptosis (Zanella *et al.*, 1999), whereas expression of *fra*-1 and c-*jun* (Timblin *et al.*, 1995) has been linked with proliferation and morphological transformation of epithelial cells (reviewed in Reddy and Mossman, 2002).

In addition to c-*fos*, the expression of several other genes associated with apoptosis is also increased in epithelial cell lines (C10) exposed to PM. The tumour necrosis factor (TNF) receptor and FAS/FAS ligand (FASL) apoptosis-related proteins are two important pathways associated with cell death. In cells (C10) exposed to PM, increases in TNF Receptor 1 (TNFR), TNFR-associated death domain (TRADD), receptor-interacting protein (RIP), Fas-associated death domain (FADD), Caspase-8, FAS and FASL mRNA levels are observed with no apparent dose-related pattern (Timblin *et al.*, 2002). This suggests that apoptosis-related gene expression is induced in epithelial cells *in vitro* by PM. However, the activity of the associated gene products and the relationship to apoptotic or surviving cells remains yet to be determined.

6.4. *NF-Kappa B*

The transcription factor NF-κB is also activated by a number of different oxidants and has been shown to regulate the expression of a number of genes involved in inflammation, cell proliferation and survival. Residual oil fly ash (ROFA), a component of PM in the USA, has been shown to activate NF-κB in a human airway epithelial cell line (BEAS-2B) and is correlated with increased expression of the pro-inflammatory genes, including those coding for the interleukins, IL-6, IL-8, and TNFα (Quay *et al.*, 1998; Kennedy *et al.*, 1998). In these studies, increased expression was ameliorated by the pre-treatment of cells with antioxidants, indicating the likely importance of ROS in these responses.

In a murine model using nose-only inhalation of ambient PM, Shukla *et al.* (2003), demonstrated increased expression of a number of cytokine genes, following a short (6 hour) period of exposure to urban $PM_{2.5}$ followed by a 24-hour recovery. In these experiments, mRNA levels of TNFα and β, IL-6, Interferon, and Transforming Growth Factor-β 1-3, were increased in mice exposed to $250\,\mu g/m^3$ air of $PM_{2.5}$, in comparison with levels in sham-exposed mouse lungs. In murine C10 pulmonary epithelial cell lines and a derived stable NF-κB-luciferase reporter cell line, exposure to ambient PM at a non-cytotoxic concentration ($10\,\mu g/cm^2$ dish) resulted in both increased binding of NF-κB to DNA and NF-κB-dependent gene expression; both were decreased in the presence of catalase. These studies also showed the early and persistent production of oxidants, measured using flow cytometry and cell laser scanning microscopy in C10 cells exposed to PM or ultrafine CB particles.

Overall, these data suggest that the exposure of pulmonary epithelial cell lines to non-cytotoxic concentrations of PM *in vitro* results in increases in c-*jun* kinase activity, levels of phosphorylated c-Jun immunoreactive protein and transcriptional activation of AP-1-dependent gene expression. These changes are accompanied by elevations in the number of cells incorporating 5'-bromodeoxyuridine, a marker of unscheduled DNA synthesis and/or cell proliferation. Data presented here are the first to demonstrate that the interaction of ambient PM with target cells of the lung initiates several signalling pathways that may lead to proliferation, apoptosis and production of cytokines; whether these are protective or detrimental effects remains an area open for debate.

7. Proteomics

Proteomics is used to separate and identify proteins in a complex mixture for the purpose of quantitative and functional analysis of all the proteins present (Hunter *et al.*, 2002). It has proven to be a powerful tool for identifying early changes at the protein level in diseases (Kvasnicka, 2002). It can also provide a non-invasive technique for evaluating body fluids in search for pertinent or specific biomarkers of toxicity (Kennedy, 2001).

Sample preparation is a key stage for adequate results using the two-dimensional sodium dodecyl sulphate polyacrylamide gel electrophoresis (2D SDS PAGE) techniques (Rabilloud, 1999; Macri *et al.*, 2000; Molloy, 2000). It is essential that there is no loss or modification of proteins from the sample. In order to avoid this, treatment of the sample should be kept to a minimum. Samples should always be kept on ice during any treatment and the sample preparation time should be kept as short as possible (Westermeir and Navan, 2003). An effective sample preparation procedure must take into account five critical considerations (Fichmann and Westermeier, 1999):

(1) Stably solubilize proteins.
(2) Prevent protein aggregation and loss of solubility during isoelectric focusing.
(3) Prevent protein.
(4) Remove or digest nucleic acids and other interfering molecules.
(5) Prevent artifactual oxidation.

7.1. *Two Dimensional SDS-PAGE*

2D SDS PAGE is the most widely used method for analysing proteins in a complex mixture. P.H. O'Farrell and J. Klose first introduced the method in 1975. 2D SDS PAGE is the combination of two separation techniques. The first dimension step is isoelectric focusing (IEF) where proteins are separated according to their charge. The second dimension is the SDS-PAGE where proteins are separated according to their molecular weight. Thousands of different proteins can be separated, with each spot on the 2D gel corresponding to a single protein species in the sample. The gels can be used to gain information such as isoelectric point, apparent molecular weight and the amount of protein obtained.

Using this technique, O'Farrell was able to resolve 1,100 different components from *Escherichia coli* and Klose-used mouse tissue to resolve 275 spots from fetal liver, with approximately 230 from whole embryos and approximately 100 for serum. Since this technique was introduced in 1975, it has been used to investigate a wide variety of samples such as normal versus disease samples, disease versus treated samples and molecular markers in body fluids (Westermeier, 2002).

7.2. *Image Analysis*

Due to the complexity of the 2D gels, it is impossible to evaluate and compare them by the human eye, requiring computer-assisted image analysis. The lack of suitable image analysis software has been a hindrance to proteomic analysis, but new software which is faster and capable of handling imperfect gels is now available. 2D expression software (Nonlinear Dynamics Ltd) is currently employed to analyse the 2D gels. The software allows the user to set up the experimental parameters and then automatically analyse the gels accordingly. The software produces a reference gel which can be used to compare any differences in spot intensities.

7.3. *Mass Spectrometry*

Mass spectrometry is used for the identification of the proteins spots separated on the 2D gels. It is a fast and highly sensitive method for providing accurate molecular weights and charges of proteins and peptides. There are two mass spectrometers currently in use: (1) Electrospray Ionization (ESI) and (2) Matrix-assisted laser desorption/ionization (MALDI). The isolated proteins are digested by trypsin to produce peptide fragments. The spectrometer measures the mass of each fragment and produces a peptide mass fingerprint. A database search (e.g. Mascot, www.matrixscience.com) is then used to identify the proteins.

7.4. *Proteomic Analysis and the Lung*

Proteomic analysis of broncho-alveolar lavage fluid (BALF) was first performed in 1979 by Bell and Hook. They used the 2D SDS PAGE technique to compile a comprehensive map of the major proteins that were present in patients suffering from pulmonary alveolar proteinosis (Bell and Hook, 1979). Soluble proteins in BAL fluid may have originated from a broad range of sources, for example, diffusion from blood across the air-blood barrier or as products from different cell types present in the lungs (Hermans *et al.*, 2003; Wattiez and Falmagne, 2005). A comparison between serum and BALF 2D protein maps revealed that a certain number of the proteins are present at a higher concentration in the BALF than in the serum, suggesting that they are specifically produced in the lungs. Hence, these proteins are good candidates for lung-specific biomarkers. They also found that these lung specific proteins could be detected in plasma using specific antibodies (Wattiez and Falmagne, 2005).

Since 1979, the technique 2D SDS PAGE has been employed by a number of research groups to investigate the changes in BALF proteins during different disease states. Lenz and co-workers compared healthy volunteers with patients suffering from idiopathic pulmonary fibrosis, sarcoidosis and asbestosis. They observed marked changes in protein spots. In particular, they found the number and intensity of low molecular weight proteins were increased in samples from diseased lungs (Lenz *et al.*, 1993).

A number of research groups have been developing master gels of BALF proteins. Noel-Georis *et al.* (2002) have comprised a database of BALF proteins in which they observed 1,200 silver stain spots, of which they could identify 900 spots as 78 different protein species. A profile of BALF proteins of patients suffering from sarcoidosis has been investigated by Sabounchi–Schutt *et al.* (2003) using proteomics. In this study, they found alterations of 21 silver stained spots, of which 17 where identified and 12 of these were found to be significantly reduced (Sabounchi–Schutt *et al.*, 2003).

7.5. *Case Study — Proteomic Analysis of Bleomycin Induced Lung Injury*

A study was undertaken to identify protein markers of oedema and inflammation. The development of pulmonary oedema is caused by a number of factors that include capillary damage and drug/chemical action (Spencer, 1985). It is also a life-threatening complication of a variety of heart and lung diseases (Roguin *et al.*, 2000).

Bleomycin has been used in a variety of animal models to induce pulmonary injury (e.g. mouse: Aso *et al.*, 1976; hamster: Starcher *et al.*, 1978 and rat: Thrall *et al.*, 1979). In this study, a double intratracheal instillation was used to investigate pulmonary injury in rats (Balharry, 2005). Bleomycin initially induces oedema and inflammation, followed by progressive destruction of the normal lung architecture

(Shen *et al.*, 1998; Balharry, 2005). BALF samples were collected seven days after the second instillation and proteomic analysis was used to compare the protein profile with BALF from saline treated rats. Preliminary results have shown the presence of the palate, lung and nasal epithelium carcinoma associated precursor protein, i.e. PLUNC (gi25282405), in BALF from bleomycin treated rats, which appears to be absent from the saline control samples. The exact biological function of this protein is unknown, however, it has been suggested to be involved in inflammatory responses to irritants in the upper airways (Bingle and Gorr, 2004).

7.6. *Other Proteomic Studies Involving BALF*

BALF and nasal lavage (NL) fluid — Lindahl *et al.* (1995) established 65% spot pattern homology. IgA and IgG were found to be significantly higher in NL fluid, possibly due to higher exposure to foreign antigens in the upper RT, compared with the lower RT.

Smokers and non-smokers — Lindahl *et al.* (1998) observed levels of IgA, ceruloplasmin and the pro form of apolipoprotein A-1 to be lower in smokers BAL fluid than in non-smokers.

Cystic fibrosis — von Bedrow *et al.* (2001) reported reduced amounts of SP-A in the BALF of cystic fibrosis. This could be due to reduced synthesis or excessive proteolytic degradation.

Interstitial lung disease — Wattiez *et al.* (2000) reported accumulation of SP-A in patients suffering from idiopathic pulmonary fibrosis. This may have been due to alterations in synthesis or release following Type II cell damage. They also found an increase in acidic low molecular weight proteins in patients suffering from idiopathic pulmonary fibrosis and hypersensitivity pneumonitis. The proteins identified were involved in cellular processing relating to proliferation.

Diesel exhaust particles — Wang *et al.* (2005) reported induction of the phosphorylation of several phosphoproteins, belonging to a number of signal and oxidative stress pathways following exposure to DEP.

Polycyclic aromatic hydrocarbons — Kim *et al.* (2004) discovered immune defence-related proteins (complement 4 and complement factor B) to be up-regulated in both automobile emission inspectors and waste incineration workers.

These studies provide potential biomarkers for a variety of lung diseases, but to date, little is known of the effects of environmental particles on lung proteomic profiles. Proteomics has the potential to provide a diagnostic test which may be applied to identify lung injury/disease caused by the inhalation of environmental particles.

8. Summary and Conclusions

Both the physical and chemical characteristics of particles should be studied when attempting to understand particle reactivity. Knowledge of these properties will help to predict their toxic potential and to relate these characteristics to the adverse health effects. It should be noted that no single technique (e.g. analytical, exposure model or, "omic") provides a complete explanation for particle-induced toxicity. Thus, a holistic approach is required, combining a range of complimentary particle collection, characterisation, toxicology and "omic" technologies.

Acknowledgements

We would like to thank the Department of Environment, Food and Rural Affairs and Natural Environment Research Council (UK), Institute for Science and Health, National Institute for Occupational Safety and Health (USA), National Heart, Lung and Blood Institute (USA), for financial support for this work.

References

Angel P. and Karin M. (1991) The role of Jun, Fos and the AP-1 complex in cell proliferation and transformation. *Biochem Biophys Acta* **1072**: 129–157.

Aso Y., Yoneda K. and Kikkawa Y. (1976) Morphologic and biochemical study of pulmonary changes induced by bleomycin in mice. *Lab Invest* **35**: 558–568.

Balharry D. (2005) *The Genomics of Lung Toxicity*. PhD Thesis, Cardiff University, Wales, UK.

Ballard S.T. and Taylor A.E. (1994) Bioelectric properties of proximal bronchiolar epithelium. *Am J Physiol* **267**(1 Pt 1): L79–L84.

Bell D.Y. and Hook G.E. (1979) Pulmonary alveolar proteinosis: Analysis of airway and alveolar proteins. *Am Rev Respir Dis* **119**(6): 979–990.

Bérubé K.A., Quinlan T.R., Moulton G., Hemenway D., O'Shaughnessey P., Vacek P. and Mossman B.T. (1996) Comparative proliferative and histopathological changes in rat lungs after inhalation of chrysotile and crocidolite asbestos. *Toxicol Appl Pharmacol* **137**: 67–74.

Bérubé K.A., Jones T.P., Williamson B.J., Winters C., Morgan A.J. and Richards R.J. (1999) Physicochemical characterization of diesel exhaust particles: Factors for assessing biological activity. *Atmos Environ* **33**(10): 1599–1614.

Bérubé K.A., Jones T.P., Sexton K. and Richards R.J. (2003a) Quantitative image analysis of urban airborne particulate matter. *Proc Roy Micro Soc* **38**(1): 3–12.

Bérubé K.A., Moreno T., Jones T.P., Richards R.J., Thomas S. and Nevalainen A. (2003b) Analysis of the chemical and biological properties of indoor air particles. In *Airborne Particles and Settled Dust in the Indoor Environment*, eds. Morawska L. and Salthammer T., WILEY-VCH, Weinhein, Germany.

Bérubé K.A., Whittaker A., Jones T.P., Moreno T. and Merolla L. (2005) London's killer smogs: How did they kill? *Proc Roy Micro Soc* **40**(3): 171–183.

Bingle C.D. and Gorr S.-U. (2004) Host defence in oral and airway epithelia: Chromosome 20 contributes a new protein family. *Int J Biochem Cell Biol* **36**: 2144–2152.

Bradford M.M. (1976) A rapid and sensitive method for the quantitation of microgram quantities of protein utilising the principle of protein-dye binding. *Anal Biochem* **72**: 248–254.

Bree L. and Cassee F.R. (2000) Toxicity of Ambient Air PM_{10}. A Critical Review of Potentially Causative Particulate Matter Properties and Mechanisms Associated with Health Effects. National Institute of Public Health and the Environment, Report Number 650010015.

Brown P.O. and Botstein D. (1999) Exploring the new world of the genome with DNA microarrays. *Nat Gen Suppl* **21**: 33–37.

Buckpitt A., Boland B., Isbell M., Morin D., Shultz M., Baldwin R., Chan K., Karlsson A., Lin C., Taff A., West J., Fanucchi M., Van Winkle L. and Plopper C. (2002) Naphthalene-induced respiratory tract toxicity: Metabolic mechanisms of toxicity. *Drug Metab Rev* **34**(4): 791–820.

Cox B., Kislinger T. and Emili A. (2005) Integrating gene and protein expression data: Pattern analysis and profile mining. *Methods* **35**(3): 303–314.

Churg A. (1996) The uptake of minerals by pulmonary cells. *Am J Respir Crit Care Med* **154**(4 Pt): 1124–1140.

Churg A. and Brauer M. (1997) Human lung parenchyma retains PM2.5. *Am J Respir Crit Care Med* **155**: 2109–2111.

Cruzan G., Carlson G.P., Johnson K.A., Andrews L.S., Banton M.I., Bevan C. and Cushman J.R. (2002) Styrene respiratory tract toxicity and mouse lung tumors are mediated by CYP2F-generated metabolites. *Regul Toxicol Pharmacol* **35**(3): 308–319.

DETR (2002) Department of Environment, Transport and the Regions. Automatic urban and rural network site information archive. http://www.aeat.co.uk/netcen/airqual.

Driscoll K.E., Carter J.M., Iype P.T., Kumari H.L., Crosby L.L., Aardema M.J., Isfort R.J., Cody D., Chestnut M.H., Burns J.L. and LeBoeuf R.A. (1995) Establishment of immortalized alveolar Type 2 epithelial cell lines from adult rats. *In Vitro Cell Dev Biol* **31**: 516–527.

Fichmann J. and Westermeier R. (1999) 2-D protein gel electrophoresis. An overview. *Meth Mol Biol* **112**: 1–7.

Flecknell P. (2002) Replacement, reduction and refinement. *ALTEX* **19**(2): 73–78.

Gilmour P.S., Brown D.M., Lindsay T.G., Beswick P.H., MacNee W. and Donaldson, K. (1996) Adverse health effects of PM_{10} particles: Involvement of iron in generation of hydroxyl radical. *Occup Environ Med* **53**: 817–822.

Green G.M. and Watson A.Y. (1995) Relation between exposure to diesel emissions and dose to the lung. In *Diesel Exhaust: A critical analysis of emissions, exposure and health effects*. Health Effects Institute, Cambridge, MA.

Greenwell L., Moreno T., Jones T.P. and Richards R.J. (2002) Particle-induced oxidative damage is ameliorated by pulmonary antioxidants. *Free Rad Biol Med* **32**(9): 898–905.

Henderson R.F., Driscoll K.E., Harkema J.R., Lindenschmidt R.C., Maples K.R. and Barr E.B. (1995) A comparison of the inflammatory response of the lung to inhaled versus instilled particles in F344 rats. *Fund App Toxicol* **24**: 183–197.

Hermans C., Dong P., Robin M., Jadoul M., Bernard A. and Bersten A.D. (2003) Determinants of serum levels of surfactant proteins A and B and Clara cell protein CC16. *Biomarkers* **8**(6): 461–471.

Ho K., Lee S., Chan Ch., Yu J., Chow J. and Yao X. (2003) Characterisation of chemical species in $PM_{2.5}$ and PM_{10} aerosols in Hong Kong. *Atmos Environ* **37**: 31–39.

Hunter T.C., Andon N.L., Koller A., Yates J.R. and Haynes P.A. (2002) The functional proteomics toolbox: Methods and applications. *J Chromatogr B Analyt Technol Biomed Life Sci* **782**(1,2): 165–181.

Janssen Y.M., Matalon S. and Mossman B.T. (1997) Differential induction of c-*fos*, c-*jun*, and apoptosis in lung epithelial cells exposed to ROS or RNS. *Am J Physiol* **273**(4 Pt 1): L789–L796.

Jones T.P., Moreno T., BéruBé K.A. and Richards R.J. (2005) Physicochemical characterisation of microscopic airborne particles from south Wales: A review of the locations and methodologies. *Sci Total Environ* **360**(1–3): 43–59.

Joris L. and Quinton P.M. (1991) Components of electrogenic transport in unstimulated equine tracheal epithelium. *Am J Physiol* **260**(6 Pt 1): L510–L515.

Kavouras I.G., Fergason S.T., Wolfson J.M. and Koutrakis P. (2000) Development and validation of a high volume low cut-off inertial impactor (HVLI). *Inhal Toxicol* **12**: 35–50.

Kavouras I.G. and Koutrakis P. (2001) Use of polyurethane foam as the impaction substrate/collection medium in conventional inertial impactors. *Aerol Sci Technol* **34**(1): 46–56.

Kennedy T., Ghio A.J., Reed W., Samet J., Zagorski J., Quay J., Carter J., Dailey L., Hoidal J. and Devlin R.B. (1998) Copper-dependent inflammation of nuclear factor kappaB activation by particulate air pollution. *Am J Respir Cell Mol Biol* **19**: 366–378.

Kennedy S. (2001) Proteomic profiling from human samples: The body fluid alternative. *Toxicol Lett* **120**(1–3): 379–384.

Kim K.M., Sangnam O., Lee J.H., Hosub I., Ryu Y.M., Oh E., Lee J., Lee E. and Sul D. (2004) Evaluation of biological monitoring markers using genomic and proteomic analysis for automobile emission inspectors and waste incinerating workers exposed to polycyclic hydrocarbons or 2,3,7,8,-tetracholrodedibenzo-p-dioxins. *Exp Mol Med* **36**(5): 396–410.

Knowles M., Murray G., Shallal J., Askin F., Ranga V., Gatzy J. and Boucher R. (1984) Bioelectric properties and ion flow across excised human bronchi. *J Appl Physiol* **56**(4): 868–877.

Kvasnicka F. (2003) Proteomics: General strategies and application to nutritionally relevant proteins. *J Chromatogr B Analyt Technol Biomed Life Sci* **787**(1): 77–89.

Lenz A.G., Meyer B., Costabel U. and Maier K. (1993) Bronchoalveolar lavage fluid proteins in human lung disease: Analysis by two-dimensional electrophoresis. *Electrophor* **14**(3): 242–244.

Lindahl M., Stahlbom B. and Tagesson C. (1995) Two-dimensional gel electrophoresis of nasal and bronchoalveolar lavage fluids after occupational exposure. *Electrophor* **16**(7): 1199–1204.

Lindahl M., Stahlbom B., Svartz J. and Tagesson C. (1998) Protein patterns of human nasal and bronchoalveolar lavage fluids analyzed with two-dimensional gel electrophoresis. *Electrophor* **19**(18): 3222–3229.

Lockhart D.J. and Winzeler E.A. (2000) Genomics, Gene Expression and DNA Arrays. *Nature* **405**: 827–836.

Malkinson A.M., Dwyer-Nield L.D., Rice P.L. and Dinsdale D. (1997) Mouse lung epithelial cell lines- tools for the study of differentiation and neoplastic phenotype. *Toxicol* **123**: 53–100.

Macri J. and Rapundalo S.T. (2001) Application of proteomics to the study of cardiovascular biology. *Trends Cardiovasc Med* **1**(2): 66–75.

Merolla L. and Richards R.J. (2005) *In vitro* effects of water-soluble metals present in UK particulate matter. *Exp Lung Res* **31**(7): 671–683.

Molloy M.P. (2000) Two-dimensional electrophoresis of membrane proteins using immobilized pH gradients *Anal Biochem* **280**(1): 1–10.

Moreno T., Gibbons W., Jones T. and Richards R.J. (2003) The geology of ambient aerosols: Characterising urban and rural/coastal silicate PM_{10} & $PM_{2.5-0.1}$ using high volume cascade collection and scanning electron microscopy. *Atmos Environ* **37**: 4265–4276.

Moreno T., Jones T.P. and Richards R.J. (2004) Aerosol particulate matter from urban and industrial environments: Examples from Cardiff and Port Talbot, South Wales, UK. *Sci Total Environ* **334–335**: 337–346.

Mossman B.T. and Churg A. (1998) Mechanisms in the pathogenesis of asbestos and silicosis. *Am J Respir Crit Care Med* **157**: 1666–1680.

Murphy S.A., BéruBé K.A., Pooley F.D. and Richards R.J. (1998) The response of lung epithelium to well characterized fine particles. *Life Sci* **62**(19): 1789–1799.

Neas E.D. and Collins M.J. (1988) *Microwave Heating: Theoretical Concepts and Equipment Design.* Kingston H.M. and Jassie L.B., eds. American Chemical Society, Washington.

Nel A. (2005) Air pollution-related illness: Effects of particles. *Science* **308**(5723): 804–806.

Noel-Georis I., Bernard A., Falmagne P. and Wattiez R. (2002) Database of bronchoalveolar lavage fluid proteins. *J Chromatogr B Analyt Technol Biomed Life Sci* **771**(1,2): 221–236.

Oberdorster G., Oberdorster E. and Oberdorster J. (2005) Nanotoxicology: An emerging discipline evolving from studies of ultrafine particles. *Environ Health Perspect* **113**(7): 823–839.

O'Farrell P.H. (1975) High resolution two-dimensional electrophoresis of proteins. *J Biol Chem* **250**(10): 4007–4021.

Osier M. and Oberdorster G. (1997) Intratracheal inhalation versus intratracheal instillation: Differences in particle effects. *Fund Appl Toxicol* **40**: 220–227.

Pagan I., Costa D.L., McGee J.K., Richards J.H. and Dye J.A. (2003) Metals mimic airway epithelial injury induced by *in vitro* exposure to Utah Valley ambient particulate matter extracts. *J Toxicol Environ Health A* **66**(12): 1087–1112.

Quay J.L., Reed W., Samet J. and Devlin R.B. (1998) Air pollution particles induce IL-6 gene expression in human airway epithelial cells via NF-κB activation. *Am J Respir Cell Mol Biol* **19**: 98–106.

Querol X., Alastuey A., Rodriguez S., Plana F., Mantilla E. and Ruiz C. (2001) Monitoring of PM_{10} and $PM_{2.5}$ around primary particulate anthropogenic emission sources. *Atmos Environ* **35**: 845–858.

Rabilloud T. (1999) Solubilization of proteins in 2-D electrophoresis. An outline. *Meth Mol Biol* **112**: 9–19.

Reddy S.P. and Mossman B.T. (2002) Role and regulation of activator protein-1 in toxicant-induced responses of the lung. *Am J Physiol Lung Cell Mol Physiol* **283**(6): L1161–L1178.

Richards R.J., Atkins J., Marrs T.C., Brown R.F.R. and Masek L. (1989) The biochemical and pathological-changes produced by intratracheal instillation of zinc hexachloroethane smoke. *Toxicol* **54**: 79–88.

Roguin A., Behar D.B., Ami H.B., Reisner S.A., Edelstein S., Linn S. and Edoute Y. (2000) Long-term prognosis of acute pulmonary oedema — an ominous outcome. *Eur J Heart Fail* **2**: 137–144.

Sabounchi-Schutt F., Astrom J., Hellman U., Eklund A. and Grunewald J. (2003) Changes in bronchoalveolar lavage fluid proteins in sarcoidosis: A proteomics approach. *Eur Respir J* **21**(3): 414–420.

Schlesinger R.B. (1985) Comparative deposition of inhaled aerosols in experimental animals and humans: A review. *J Toxicol Environ Health* **15**(2): 197–214.

Schwartz J. and Neas L.M. (2000) Fine particles are more strongly associated than coarse particles with acute respiratory health effects in schoolchildren. *Epidemiol* **11**(1): 6–10.

Shen A.S., Haslett C., Feldsien D.C., Henson P.M. and Cherniack R.M. (1988) The intensity of chronic lung inflammation and fibrosis after bleomycin is directly related to the severity of acute injury. *Am Rev Respir Dis* **137**: 564–571.

Shukla A., Timblin C., BéruBé K.A., Gordon T., McKinney W., Driscoll K., Vacek P. and Mossman B.T. (2000) Inhaled particulate matter causes expression of nuclear factor (NF)-κb-related genes and oxidant dependent NF-κb activation *in vitro*. *Am J Resp Cell Mol Biol* **23**: 182–187.

Spencer H. (1985) Pulmonary Oedema and Its Complications and the Effects of Some Toxic Gases and Substances on the Lung. In *Pathology of the Lung*, Pergamon, New York.

Starcher B.C., Kuhn C. and Overton J.E. (1978) Increased elastin and collagen content in the lungs of hamsters receiving an intratracheal injection of bleomycin. *Am Rev Respir Dis* **117**: 299–305.

Stohs S.J. and Bagchi D. (1995) Oxidative mechanisms in the toxicity of metal ions. *Free Rad Biol Med* **18**(2): 321–336.

Thrall R.S., McCormick J.R., Jack R.M., McReynolds R.A. and Ward P.A. (1979) Bleomycin induced pulmonary fibrosis in the rat. *Am J Pathol* **95**: 117–130.

Timblin C., Janssen Y. and Mossman B.T. (1995) Transcriptional activation of the proto-oncogene c-jun by asbestos and H_2O_2 is directly related to increased proliferation and transformation of tracheal epithelial cells. *Cancer Res* **55**: 2723–2726.

Timblin C., BéruBé K.A., Churg A., Driscoll K., Gordon T., Hemenway D., Walsh E., Cummins A.B., Vacek P. and Mossman B.T. (1998) Ambient particulate matter causes activation of the *c-jun* kinase/stress-activated protein kinase cascade and DNA synthesis in lung epithelial cells. *Cancer Res* **58**: 4543–4547.

Urbanski N.K. and Beresewicz A. (2000) Generation of •OH initiated by interaction of Fe^{2+} and Cu^+ with dioxygen; comparison with the Fenton chemistry. *Acta Biochim Pol* **47**(4): 951–962.

von Bedrow *et al.* (2001) Surfactant protein A and other bronchoalveolar lavage fluid proteins are altered in cystic fibrosis. *Eur Respir J* **17**(4): 716–722.

Wang M., Xiao G.G., Li N., Xie Y., Loo J.A. and Nel A.E. (2005) Use of a fluorescent phosphoprotein dye to characterize oxidative stress-induced signaling pathway components in macrophage and epithelial cultures exposed to diesel exhaust particle chemicals. *Electrophor* **11**: 2092–2108.

Noel-Georis I., Bernard A., Falmagne P. and Wattiez R. (2002) Database of bronchoalveolar lavage fluid proteins. *J Chromatogr B Analyt Technol Biomed Life Sci* **771**(1,2): 221–236.

Wattiez R. and Falmagne P. (2005) Proteomics of bronchoalveolar lavage fluid. *J Chromatogr B Analyt Technol Biomed Life Sci* **815**(1,2): 169–178.

Westermeir R. and Navan T. (2002) *Proteomics in Practice: A Laboratory Manual of Proteome Analysis*, Wiley-VCH, Weinheim.

Whittaker A.G. (2003) Black smokes: Past and present. Ph.D. Thesis, Cardiff University, Wales, UK.

Whittaker A., Jones T.P., BéruBé K.A., Maynard R. and Richards R.J. (2004) Killer smogs of the 1950s London: Composition of the particles and their bioactivity. *Sci Total Environ* **334–335**: 435–445.

Wilson M.R., Lightbody J.H., Donaldson K., Sales J. and Stone V. (2002) Interactions between ultrafine particles and transition metals. *Toxicol Appl Pharmacol* **184**: 172–179.

Wolz L., Krause G., Scherer G., Aufderheide M. and Mohr U. (2002) *In vitro* genotoxicity assay of sidestream smoke using a human bronchial epithelial cell line. *Food Chem Toxicol* **40**(6): 845–850.

Yang K.X., Swami K. and Husain L. (2002) Determination of trace metals in atmospheric aerosols with a heavy matrix of cellulose by microwave digestion-inductively coupled plasma mass spectroscopy. *Spectrochimica Acta* (Part B), **57**: 73–84.

Zanella C.L., Timblin C.R., Cummins A., Jung M., Goldberg J., Raabe R., Tritton T.R. and Mossman B.T. (1999) Asbestos-induced phosphorylation of epidermal growth factor receptor is linked to c-fos and apoptosis. *Am J Physiol* **277**(4 Pt 1): L684–L693.

Abbreviations

PM	Particulate Matter
PM_{10}	Mass concentration of particles generally less than 10 microns in aerodynamic diameter
$PM_{2.5}$	Mass concentration of particles of generally less than 2.5 microns aerodynamic diameter
HR-TEM	High Resolution Transmission Electron Microscopy
FESEM	Field Emission Scanning Electron Microscopy
EPXMA	Electron Probe X-ray Micro-Analysis
IA	Image Analysis
ICP-MS	Inductively Coupled Plasma Mass Spectrometry
ESD	Equivalent Spherical Diameter
PUF	Polyurethane Foam
IC	Ion Chromatography
SW	South West
SE	South East

NE	North East
NW	North West
EOCC	Elemental organic carbon compounds
PPM	Parts per million
PPT	Parts per trillion
BS	Black Smoke
ALI	Air-Liquid Interface
LM	Light Microscopy
TEER	Transepithelial Electrical Resistance
MTT-100	Mitochondrial Toxicity Assay (MatTek™)
PBS	Phosphate Buffered Saline
PCR	Polymerase Chain Reaction
RT	Reverse Transcription
CV	Coefficient of Variation
TSC	Tobacco Smoke Components
cDNA	Complementary DNA
gDNA	Genomic DNA
mRNA	Messenger RNA
MM	Metal Mixtures
PCR	Polymerase Chain Reaction
BEAS-2B	SV40 T antigen-transformed human epithelial cell line
CB	Carbon Black
C10	Murine Alveolar Type 2 cell line
RLE	Rat Lung Epithelial cell line
AP-1	Activator Protein–1
NF-κB	Nuclear Factor-kappa B
ROS	Reactive Oxygen Species
JNK	c-Jun Kinase/Stress-activated protein kinase
RLE-6TN	Rat Alveolar Type 2 Epithelial cell line
TNF	Tumour Necrosis Factor
ROFA	Residual Oil Fly Ash
2D SDS PAGE	Two-Dimensional Sodium Dodecyl Sulphate Polyacrylamide Gel Electrophoresis
IEF	Isoelectric Focusing
ESI	Electrospray Ionization
MALDI	Matrix-assisted laser desorption/ionization
BALF	Broncho-alveolar Lavage Fluid

CHAPTER 5

ACID AEROSOLS AS
A HEALTH HAZARD

Lung Chi Chen, George Thurston and
Richard B. Schlesinger

1. Introduction

A key consideration in the evaluation of PM-health effects is whether
there are specific chemical components of PM that are responsible
for some or all of the noted epidemiological associations between PM
and adverse human health outcomes. The presence of known toxic
constituents within ambient particles would add to the plausibility of
these associations. This chapter considers the effect of aerosol acidity,
based on epidemiological, toxicological and human clinical studies.
This will allow the development of conclusions as to exposure concentrations and duration that may be associated with adverse health
effects and whether exposure conditions exist, which would likely be
a cause for concern in terms of public health, due to exposure to
ambient PM.

2. Formation of Atmospheric Acid Aerosols

The major source of particulate phase acidity is the atmospheric transformation of SO_2, with 20% of emitted SO_2 undergoing conversion.
This reaction may occur in the gas phase (homogeneous gas-phase
reaction), on the surface of other atmospheric particles (heterogeneous gas-solid reaction), or within atmospheric aqueous droplets

(homogeneous liquid-phase reaction) following a heterogeneous gas-solid reaction, and results in the production of SO_3, which then combines with water vapor, producing sulphuric acid particles. Since many particles already exist in the polluted environment to interact with acids formed from pollutant gases such as sulphur oxides, heterogeneous nucleation is the most common formation pathway (e.g. see NRC, 1977). Thus, acidic aerosols are not usually formed by homogeneous nucleation, and are not usually present in the ambient air as pure acid aerosols.

The secondarily produced acid aerosol generally does not remain strongly acidic in the atmosphere for extended periods of time, since it will eventually be partially or completely neutralized by atmospheric ammonia (NH_3). Pure sulphuric acid, often used as the model for acidic sulphates in toxicological studies, rarely exists in ambient outdoor air, and the acidic sulphate component usually consists of ammonium bisulphate, or a mixture of sulphuric acid, with partially to completely neutralized sulphates, in combination with other particulate mass with which the acid usually co-exists. The toxicity of this other particulate matter may be influenced by the co-presence of the acid (e.g. as a surface coating, or in aerosol solution), including the lowering of its pH, and potential increases in the solubility and bio-availabilty of some PM components, such as particulate transition metals that may be involved in oxidative stress (Costa and Dreher, 1997). Thus, assessments of the toxicity of ambient acidic aerosols must consider both the direct and indirect effects of the acidity on particle toxicity.

3. Exposure Levels

In North America, regional air pollution episodes generally occur in the summer time and are characterised by high sulphate concentrations occurring over hours to days, often in association with secondary oxidant pollutants such as ozone. Local plume impacts involve exposures all year and occur downwind of strong point sources such as power plants or smelters. Acid fogs are associated with cool temperatures and they result from the condensation of water vapour on preexisting fine particles (diameter $< 10\,\mu m$) when the atmosphere is saturated (i.e. RH $= 100\%$).

In the USA, seasonal peaks of sulphuric acid at $0.02–0.04\,\text{mg/m}^3$ occur, but annual averages are generally $< 0.005\,\text{mg/m}^3$ (Lioy and Waldman, 1989). No country has an ambient air quality standard specifically for acid aerosols, when it is regarded as part of the general particulate matter standards.

4. Dosimetry and Fate

Inhaled sulphate aerosols will deposit in the respiratory tract depending on specific aerosol particle size distribution and host ventilation characteristics as with any aerosol. However, sulphate particles may alter their size following inhalation, due to deliquescence (e.g. ammonium bisulphate) or hygroscopicity (e.g. sulphuric acid), which may result in a substantial growth in diameter, often by factors of 2–4 times within the airways. Such particles will then deposit on airway surfaces according to their hydrated rather than their initial dry size (Morrow, 1986; Martonen and Zhang, 1993).

Inhaled sulphate particles may also be partly neutralized by respiratory tract ammonia (Larson *et al.*, 1977; Larson *et al.*, 1982), particularly with oral inhalation. Deposited acid sulphate particles may be further modified by buffering in the fluid lining of the airways (Holma, 1985).

The extent of reaction between acid particles and respiratory tract ammonia depends on a number of factors (Larson, 1993). Neutralisation is inversely proportional to particle size within the relevant ambient diameter range of $0.1–10\,\mu\text{m}$. Different combinations of ammonia and ventilation rates result in lesser or greater amounts of acidic sulphates becoming available for deposition, even with constant inhaled acid concentration.

5. Health Effects of Acidic Aerosols

5.1. *Epidemiological Evidence*

Acid aerosol health effects during pollution episodes

Some of the earliest effects of ambient acid aerosols on human health stem from historically important air pollution episodes, such as those in the Meuse Valley (Belgium), Donora, PA (USA), and London (UK).

The episodes in the Meuse Valley in 1930 resulted in more than 60 deaths, the mortality rate during the fog being more than ten times higher than the usual. Those persons especially affected were the elderly, i.e. those suffering from asthma, heart patients and the debilitated (Firket, 1931). Sulphuric acid was thought to be the main causal agent.

In the Donora event of 1948, 18 deaths were attributed to the fog (Schrenk *et al.*, 1949). Examination of the water soluble fraction of solids on a filter of an electronic air cleaner operating during the smog suggested that acid particles were an important component (Hemeon, 1955).

During the London fog of December 1952, apart from considerable respiratory symptomatology, at least 4,000 excess deaths from respiratory and cardiovascular conditions occurred. The UK Ministry of Health (United Kingdom Ministry of Health, 1954) report concluded that: "It is probable, therefore, that sulphur trioxide dissolved as sulphuric acid in fog droplets, appreciably reinforced the harmful effects."

Acid aerosol data from the December 1962 London Fog episode provided some of the strongest evidence that acid aerosols were elevated during the 1950s episodes (Commins and Waller, 1967). 24-hour average acid concentrations reached $378\,\mu g/m^3$ (as H_2SO_4) on the peak mortality day during this latter event, although both Black Smoke and SO_2 were also elevated, so a single causal factor could not be identified.

Both mortality and morbidity effects can be associated with pollutant mixes which include elevated levels of acid aerosols. The calculations and measurements of sulphuric acid levels (estimated to range up to $678\,\mu g/m^3$ for a 1-hour average) during some London episodes in the late 50s and early 60s provide a plausible basis for hypothesising contributions of sulphuric acid aerosols to the health effects observed during those episodes.

Quantitative analyses of London mortality and daily acid aerosols

Reanalysis of the London mortality data from the 1960s and 70s provided further insight into the role of aerosol acid and health effects. Thurston *et al.* (1989) found that the log of sulphuric acid measured at the central site was much more strongly correlated with raw total daily mortality than any measure of BS or SO_2, especially with a 1-day lag ($r = 0.31$), more so when the data were log transformed. However, allowance for temporal trends weakened the correlation of H_2SO_4 with raw total mortality [e.g. $r = 0.19$ for log (H_2SO_4) with next day filtered mortality].

Subsequently, a more extensive analysis of the London total mortality and acid aerosol data was conducted for 1965 to 1972, using year round daily acid measurements (for methodological details see Ito *et al.*, 1993). Significant associations with same day and following days' mortality were found for H_2SO_4, SO_2 and BS. In the most extensively controlled model, the winter mean pollutant effect was estimated to range from 2 to 3% of the mean 278 deaths/day total mortality, but all three pollutants gave similar results (for mean $H_2SO_4 = 5.0\,\mu g/m^3$, $SO_2 = 293\,\mu g/m^3$, or BS $= 72\,\mu g/m^3$), but their respective effects could not be separated due to their high inter-correlation. These models fit well to the (separate) 1962 London acid/mortality episode data, supporting the validity of such deviation-derived mortality estimates.

A different approach analysed restricted temperature ranges in each season (Lippmann and Ito, 1995). In each season, the majority of days fell within one or two temperature ranges, within which the mortality also fell within narrow ranges. Within these restricted ranges, analyses indicated that there were relatively strong associations between daily mortality and the daily logs of the concentrations of hydrogen ion (H^+) and SO_2 (see Fig. 1), but not with BS. While attractive, this approach does not address the need to control for the potential effects of prior days' extreme temperatures (i.e. lagged effects), nor are the potential temperature effects within the ranges considered. The most interesting result of these analyses is probably that the H^+-mortality association is found even in the summertime, when the daily H^+ concentrations do not exceed approximately $10\,\mu g/m^3$, as H_2SO_4 (~ 200 nmoles H^+/m^3).

Acute acidic aerosol exposure studies of children

As part of the 6-Cities study conducted by Harvard University, a cohort of approximately 1,800 school children from six U.S. cities

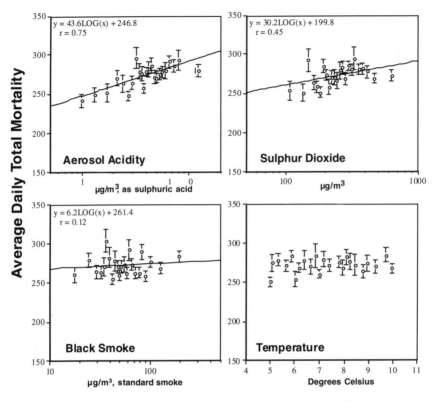

Fig. 1. Plots of average daily mortality in greater London versus temperature and log of pollutant concentrations for winter days (1965–1972) having ambient temperatures between 5 and 10 degrees celsius (Lippmann and Ito, 1995).

was enrolled in a diary study in which parents completed a bi-weekly report on each child's daily respiratory symptoms (Schwartz *et al.*, 1994). Analyses of daily lower respiratory symptoms (LRS) found, in individual pollutant regressions, that PM_{10}, $PM_{2.5}$, $PM_{2.5}$ sulphur (i.e. sulphates), nephelometry (an index of sub-micron particle concentration), SO_2, and ozone O_3 were all significant predictors. Of these, $PM_{2.5}$ sulphur (i.e. sulphates) and PM_{10} yielded the highest levels of significance suggesting that the sulphur containing fine aerosol component was driving the PM relationships found with LRS. In the overall data analysis, aerosol acidity was not significantly associated with LRS, but associations were noted for H^+ above 110 nmoles/m³, with a relative odds ratio of LRS estimated to be greater than 2.0 at 300 nmoles/m^3 H$^+$. Similarly, upper respiratory symptoms showed no consistent association with H$^+$ until concentrations exceeded 110 nmoles/m^3. The exposure-dependent increase in symptoms seen across the entire range of PM$_{10}$ suggests that the effect is principally related to particle mass, but the results also suggest that the presence of acid may increase the particulate effect, if it is in high enough concentrations.

A separate, limited analysis of upper respiratory symptoms employing continuously monitored H$_2$SO$_4$ data, rather than H$^+$ measured from filter samples, showed that the largest regression coefficient for these symptoms was with H$_2$SO$_4$, the strongest association falling on the first two days (Schwartz *et al.*, 1991).

In a study of ambient air pollution and lung function in children (Neas *et al.*, 1995), a sample of 83 children living in Uniontown, PA, performed twice daily peak expiratory flow (PEF) measurements and recorded symptoms on 3,582 child-days during the summer of 1990. These were analysed in relation to ambient temperature, O$_3$, SO$_2$, fine particle mass, PM$_{10}$, and H$^+$. A 12-hour exposure to a 125 nmole/m^3 increment in H$^+$ was associated with a -2.5 liters/minute deviation in the group mean PEF (95% CI = -4.2 to -0.8) and with increased cough incidence (odds ratio, OR = 1.6; 95% CI = 1.1 to 2.4), although H$^+$ was highly correlated with sulphates (r = 0.92) and fine particles (r = 0.86). A 30 ppb increment in 12-hour ozone was associated with a similar deviation in PEF (OR = -2.8; 95% CI = -6.7 to 1.1). When both O$_3$ and H$^+$ were entered into the model simultaneously, the H$^+$ effect size was only slightly reduced and remained significant. Although monitored, PM$_{10}$ results were not presented for comparison. Thus, summertime occurrences of elevated acid aerosol and particulate sulphate pollution are associated with acute, albeit small declines in PEF and increased incidence of cough episodes in children.

A study of winter-type pollution and asthmatics was conducted in Erfurt and Weimar, Germany, and the Czech Republic city of Sokolov from September, 1990 through June, 1992 (Peters *et al.*, 1996). A panel of 155 children and 102 adults with asthma recorded daily symptoms, medication intake, and PEF. Weak same-day effects and a stronger cumulative effect of air pollution was observed for both PEF and for symptoms in children, but less so in adults. The 5-day mean of aerosol acidity was significantly correlated with a decrease in PEF in children (an interquartile range change of $0.42\,\mu g/m^3$ was associated with a -0.52% change in PEF (95% CI $= -0.89$–0.16, t $= -2.82$), but not as strongly as SO_2 or sulphate. Regressions with more than one pollutant were not reported, but it was mentioned that H^+ varied relatively independently of the other pollutants (e.g. $r^2 = 0.18$ with PM_{10} in Sokolov), which may indicate that its association with PEF is distinct from that of the other pollutants. The H^+ levels were lower than expected in these high SO_2 areas, suggesting that morbidity in children was best predicted by SO_2 and SO_4.

The low H^+ levels recorded in these high SO_2 cities were thought to be due to neutralisation by ammonia (Brauer *et al.*, 1995), but sample neutralisation by alkaline fine particles may have contributed to it as well. As shown in Table 1, the ion balance in both of these cities was off by 5 to 11%, with the cations being under-represented relative to the anions. This is expected to be the case if some of the acids were being neutralised on the filter by alkaline fine particles, thereby causing the measured H^+ to be spuriously lower. While 5 to 11% does not sound large, this is the percentage of the entire amount of anions, much bigger than the amount of H^+. Thus, if this ion balance difference is due to artifactual loss of H^+, the actual atmospheric H^+ is much higher than that which is measured from the filter. In this case, it can be seen in Table 1 that, after considering the cations unaccounted for by the ion balance, the potential underestimation of H^+ (and the associated errors in measurement introduced) can be quite large, with the maximum possible mean H^+ concentrations in these cities being two to five times as large as measured on the filter.

Overall, most of these paediatric studies provide evidence consistent with an acute acidic PM effect on both children's respiratory function and symptoms. However, given the usually high correlation between H^+ and PM mass in these studies, it is difficult to discriminate those effects solely related to the acid portion of PM.

Table 1. Summary statistics for denuder/filter pack measurements of PM species made in Sokolov, Czech Republic and Erfurt, Germany (Brauer *et al.*, 1995) with adjustments to H^+ based on anion-cation imbalance (nanoequivalents/m^3).

Site	Mean H$^+$ raw (Teflon filter)	Mean H$^+$ corr.*	Mean SO$_4^=$ (Teflon filter)	Mean NO$_3^-$ (Teflon filter)	Total Anions (Teflon filter) Site	Cation/ Anion Ratio	Missing Cation	Maximum Possible Mean H$^+$
Sokolov	13.6	15.9	198.6	51.9	250.5	0.95	12.5	28.4
Erfurt	8.9	12.9	219.4	48.8	268.2	0.89	29.5	42.4

*H$^+$corr. = Acid aerosol concentration after correction for acid losses due to reactions with ammonium nitrate on the filter.

Acute acid aerosol exposure studies of adults

The hypothesis that human exposures to ambient H^+ concentrations are associated with exacerbations of pre-existing respiratory disease was tested by a recent study of responses to airborne acid aerosols in asthmatics (Ostro *et al.*, 1991). Daily concentrations of aerosol H^+, $SO_4^=$, NO_3, and FP, SO_2 and HNO_3 (but not CO or NO_2), were correlated with daily symptom, medication usage, and other variables for a panel of 207 adults with moderate to severe asthma in Denver between November 1987 and March 1988. The H^+ concentrations ranged from 2 to 41 neq/m^3 (0.01 to 2.0 μg/m^3 of H_2SO_4 equivalent), and were significantly related to both the proportion of the survey respondents reporting a moderate or worse overall asthma condition, and the proportion reporting a moderate or worse cough. However, these concentrations are near to or below the level of detection of H^+, and of the 74 H^+ values used in the analysis, 47 were predicted from the observed $SO_4^=$ value on that day (H^+-$SO_4^=$ correlation = 0.66), which is more accurately measured at such low levels. PM$_{2.5}$ was also highly correlated with sulphates during this study (r = 0.86). Both logit models and ordinary least squares with a log pollution term, autoregressive terms, and terms for trend, weekend, use of gas stove, and maximum daily temperature were modelled.

For asthma, elasticities (the percent change in the health effect due to a given percent change in the pollutant) with respect to $SO_4^=$, FP, and H^+ were 0.060, 0.055 and 0.096, respectively (Ostro *et al.*, 1991), indicating that a doubling of the concentration of H^+ (from 8 to 16 nmoles/m^3) would increase the proportion reporting a moderate to severe asthma condition by 10%. When examined for evidence of lagged effects, contemporaneous measures of H^+ concentration provided the best associations with asthma status, and that meteorological variables were not associated with the health effects reported. After adjusting for time spent outdoors, level of activity, and penetration of acid aerosol indoors, the effect of H^+ on cough increased 43%, suggesting that dose-response estimates that do not incorporate behavioural factors affecting actual H^+ exposures may substantially underestimate the impact of the pollution. While these results allow the consideration that human exposures to present day ambient H^+ concentrations may be associated with exacerbations of pre-existing respiratory disease, the H^+ concentrations on some days had to be estimated from sulphate levels, and potentially confounding pollutants were not simultaneously considered with H^+ in the model.

Acute acidic aerosol associations with respiratory hospital admissions

Thurston *et al.* (1992) analysed unscheduled (emergency) admissions to acute care hospitals in three New York State metropolitan areas during the summers of 1988 and 1989, including one site (NYC) located well outside the urban core (in White Plains, 10 mi. north of the city), where acid levels are likely to be overestimates of the levels experienced directly in the city. However, comparisons between sulphates in the White Plains site and at a site in Manhattan during part of the study period showed a high correlation ($r = 0.9$), supporting the assumption that the White Plains H^+ data are indicative of particulate strong acid exposures in NYC. The strongest pollutant-respiratory admissions associations found by Thurston *et al.* (Gwynn *et al.*, 2000) were during the high pollution 1988 summer, and in the most urbanised communities. Correlations between the pollution data and hospital admissions for non-respiratory control diseases were non-significant both before and after prefiltering. After controlling for temperature effects via simultaneous regression, the summer haze pollutants (i.e. $SO_4^=$, H^+, and O_3) remained significantly related to total respiratory and asthma admissions. However, multiple pollutant regressions were not attempted, preventing a clear discrimination of these pollutants respective effects. Other pollutants were not considered, but were generally low and unlikely to be highly correlated with the studied pollutants during July and August in these cities. After filtering, $SO_4^=$ and H^+ were highly correlated in these cities (e.g. $r = 0.86$ in Buffalo, and 0.79 in NYC during the summer of 1988), supporting the contention that SO_4 is a useful index of H^+ in these time-series analyses. In regressions for the summer of 1988 for Buffalo and New York City, both H^+ and $SO_4^=$ had similar mean effects (3 to 4% of respiratory admissions in NYC, at mean $H^+ = 2.4\,\mu g/m^3$ as H_2SO_4, and mean $SO_4^= = 9.3\,\mu g/m^3$; and 6 to 8% in Buffalo, at mean $H^+ = 2.2\,\mu g/m^3$

as H_2SO_4, and mean $SO_4^= = 9.0\,\mu g/m^3$). Ozone mean effects estimates were always larger than H^+ or $SO_4^=$, but the impact of the
highest day was greatest for H^+ in all cases. This is the case in part
because H^+ episodes are more extreme, relative to the mean, than
are O_3 episodes (e.g. in Buffalo in 1988, the summer max./mean
$H^+ = 8.5$, while the max./mean $O_3 = 2.2$). Thus, the H^+ effects estimates reported in this work are dominated by the two or three peak
H^+ days per year experienced in these cities (e.g. $H^+ > 10\,\mu g/m^3$,
or $\sim 200\,\text{nmoles}/m^3$, as a 24-hour average).

A study of respiratory hospital admissions in the Toronto
metropolitan area during the summers of 1986 to 1988 (Thurston
et al., 1994) was designed specifically to test the hypothesis that the
$SO_4^=$ associations previously found in Southern Ontario were due
to H^+ exposures. Strong and significant positive associations with
both asthma and respiratory admissions were found for both O_3 and
H^+, as well as somewhat weaker significant associations with $SO_4^=$. No
such associations were found for SO_2 or NO_2, nor for any pollutant
with non-respiratory control admissions. Other PM metrics examined
included the mass of fine particles less than 2.5 mm in d_a (FP), the
mass of particles greater than 2.5 μm and less than 10 μm in d_a (CP),
PM_{10} (= FP + CP), TSP, and non-thoracic TSP (= TSP-PM_{10}). Temperature was only weakly correlated with respiratory admissions, and
became non-significant when entered in regressions with air pollution indices.

Of these pollutants, only H^+ remained significant in the respiratory admissions regression when both O_3 and temperature were
also included (see Table 2). Furthermore, the correlation of the H^+
and O_3 coefficients in this simultaneous model was non-significant
($r = -0.11$), indicating that these two pollutants have independent
associations with respiratory admissions. The 1988 results for Toronto
were consistent with those found previously for nearby Buffalo, NY
(approximately 100 km to the south, across Lake Ontario). As in
the Buffalo analysis, the maximum H^+ day in Toronto (August 4,
1988: $H^+ = 391\,\text{nmoles}/m^3$) showed the greatest relative risk of
total respiratory and asthma admissions (1.50 and 1.53, respectively),
again indicating an especially large adverse respiratory effect by
summertime haze air pollutants during the few H^+ episode days each

Table 2. Simultaneous regressions of 1986–1988 toronto daily summertime total respiratory admissions on temperature and various pollution metrics (Thurston *et al.*, 1994b).

Temp., Pollutant Model Specification	Pollutant Regr. Coefficients (adm/poll. unit*)	*p*-value (one-way)
Single Pollutant Models:		
T(LG0), O_3 (LG0)	0.0528 ± 0.0197	0.004
T(LG0), H^+ (LG0)	0.0227 ± 0.0096	0.010
T(LG0), $SO_4^=$ (LG0)	0.0106 ± 0.0054	0.028
T(LG0), FP(LG0)	0.0828 ± 0.0367	0.013
T(LG0), CP(LG0)	0.1228 ± 0.0895	0.086
T(LG0), PM_{10}(LG0)	0.0642 ± 0.0290	0.015
T(LG0), TSP(LG0)	0.0242 ± 0.0160	0.066
T(LG0), TSP-PM_{10}(LG0)	0.0180 ± 0.0196	0.180
Two Pollutant Models:		
T(LG0), O_3 (LG0)	0.0503 ± 0.0205	0.008
H_+(LG1)	0.0153 ± 0.0089	0.044
T(LG0), O_3 (LG0)	0.0508 ± 0.0207	0.008
$SO_4^=$(LG1)	0.0062 ± 0.0046	0.089
T(LG0), O_3 (LG0)	0.0404 ± 0.0233	0.043
FP(LG0)	0.0434 ± 0.0429	0.157
T(LG0), O_3 (LG0)	0.0388 ± 0.0241	0.055
PM_{10}(LG0)	0.0339 ± 0.0344	0.164
T(LG0), O_3 (LG0)	0.0360 ± 0.0228	0.059
TSP(LG0)	0.0127 ± 0.0175	0.235

*Pollution units are nmoles/m^3 for H^+ and $SO_4^=$, ppb for O_3, and $\mu g/m^3$ for FP, CP, PM_{10}, TSP, and TSP-PM_{10}.

summer. However, a sensitivity analysis eliminating the six days having $H^+ \geq 100$ nmoles/m^3 yielded a similar and statistically significant H^+ coefficient in the total respiratory admissions regression, suggesting that the association is not limited to the highest pollution days. The authors concluded that the associations between summertime haze air pollutants (i.e. O_3 and H^+) and acute exacerbations of respiratory disease (i.e. respiratory hospital admissions) were causal. It is of particular interest to note that, assuming the H^+ to be in the form of

NH_4HSO_4, the "effect" per $\mu g/m^3$ of mass implied by these Toronto coefficients indicate that H^+ is six times as potent (per $\mu g/m^3$) as the non-acidic components of PM_{10}.

The studies of daily respiratory hospital admissions in New York State cities and in Toronto, Ontario support the hypothesis that the summertime sulphate concentrations are accompanied by acidic aerosols in Eastern North America and that the H^+ associations with respiratory hospital admissions were found to be stronger than for sulphates, or any other PM component monitored. The facts that: (1) these were studies designed specifically to test the hypothesis that H^+ is associated with increased respiratory hospital admissions; (2) consistent results were found, both qualitatively and quantitatively across these studies; and (3) in one of them, many other pollutants and PM metrics were directly inter-compared with H^+ in the analyses, collectively indicate that these studies provide evidence that acid aerosols may represent a component of PM that is particularly associated with increases in the incidence of exacerbations in pre-existing respiratory disease.

Acute acid aerosol exposure associations with mortality

Relatively long records of daily mortality and pollution are required to have sufficient power to discern mortality-pollution associations. Due to the dearth of sufficiently long records of H^+ concentration measurements (other than the historical London measurements), few studies have yet attempted to evaluate the acute mortality effects of acidic aerosols.

Dockery *et al.* (1992) investigated the relationship between multiple air pollutants and total daily mortality between September 1985 and August 1986 in two communities, St. Louis, MO, Kingston/Harriman, TN and the surrounding counties. In each study area, total daily mortality was related to PM_{10}, $PM_{2.5}$, SO_2, NO_2, O_3, $SO_4^=$, H^+, temperature, dew point, and season using autoregressive Poisson models. In St. Louis, after controlling for weather and season, statistically significant associations were found with both prior day's PM_{10} and $PM_{2.5}$, but not with any lags of the other pollutants considered. In the Kingston/Harriman vicinity, PM_{10} and $PM_{2.5}$ approached significance in the mortality regression, while the other pollutants did not. In both cities, very similar PM_{10} coefficients were reported, implying around a 1.6% increase in total mortality per $10\,\mu g/m^3$ of PM_{10}. The chief areas of concern regarding this study relate to the exposure data as in both places, only one daily monitoring station was employed to represent community exposure levels, and no information regarding the representativeness of these sites were provided. More importantly in the case of H^+ analyses, the number of days for which pollution data are available for time-series analyses is very limited in this data set with much missing data. These issues limit the value of this study.

Later analysis of the entire Six Cities dataset uses time-series methods to look at short-term associations between daily mortality and air pollution. This combined analysis of the association between fine and coarse particle measurements in six US cities suggests that ambient fine particle exposures, and not coarse particle exposures, are specifically responsible for the observed associations with daily mortality. In these analyses, acid aerosols were more weakly associated with daily mortality than sulphates and fine particles. However, the numbers of H^+ measurements were one fifth of the number of observations of the other PM metrics (e.g. only 1621 for H^+, versus 8,409 for sulphates). Adjusting the H^+ t-statistics upward to account for this indicates that a significant effect on mortality would have been found (RR = 1.012 for a $67.3\,nmole/m^3$ increase, t = 1.73) had as many measurements been available for H^+ as for other metrics, although such extrapolations need to be viewed with caution. It is also worth noting that approximately one third of the H^+ data considered were below the H^+ detection limit in this dataset, indicating that a great deal of random variation was present in the dataset. An alternative to the analysis done would be to follow the procedure used by Ostro *et al.* (1991), who estimated a $SO_4^=$-H^+ relationship from days above detection, and used this relationship to predict H^+ from $SO_4^=$ measurements on days when H^+ was below detection. Also, as will be discussed later, H^+ measurements in industrialized cities like St. Louis and Steubenville may be subject to increased errors, if alkaline fine particles are collected on the filters. Overall, this study indicates that, of the PM components, fine particles and sulphates were more significantly associated with daily mortality than H^+ in the Six City dataset, but the number and quality of the H^+ data available for this analysis were less than that for fine particle or sulphates.

Gwynn *et al.* (2000) considered a much more extensive two-and-a-half year record of daily H^+ measurements (May 1988-October 1990) collected in the Buffalo, NY region in a time-series analysis of total and respiratory daily mortality and hospital admissions. Of the pollutants considered, H^+ was most consistently associated ($p < 0.05$) with adverse health effects (see Fig. 2). Relative risks (RR's) were estimated for increases equal to the maximum minus the mean concentration (e.g. 345 nmoles/m^3 for H^+, 65 μg/m^3 for PM_{10}). Respiratory hospital admissions RR estimates associated with H^+ ranged from 1.30--1.50, while those for respiratory mortality ranged from 1.48–1.60. Total mortality RR estimates for H^+ ranged from 1.14–1.17, while those for PM_{10} ranged from 1.07 to 1.08. Simultaneous regression with gaseous air pollutants had minimal effects on the H^+ RR's,

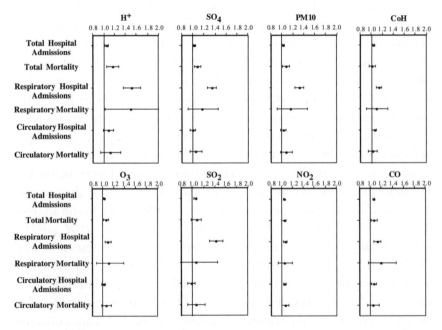

Fig. 2.   Total and underlying cause-specific relative risks (95% CI) associated with max.-mean pollutant increments for the Buffalo, NY Area, 1988–1990 (Gwynn *et al.*, 1997).

indicating that H^+ can be a significant contributor to the recorded acute adverse health effects.

Lippmann *et al.* (2000) investigated PM effects on all cause and disease specific mortality and morbidity by considering the multiple PM components in Detroit, focusing primarily on two study periods in which multiple PM components were measured: 1985 to 1990, when levels of TSP, sulphate from TSP (TSP-$SO_4^=$), PM_{10}, and non-thoracic TSP (TSP-PM_{10}) were measured throughout the year; and 1992 to 1994, when data on PM_{10}, $PM_{2.5}$, $PM_{10-2.5}$ (the coarse fraction), particle acidity (H^+), and artifact-free sulphates ($SO_4^=$) were available for mostly summer months. Overall, it was found that sulphate and the H^+ associations with mortality were weaker than for other PM metrics, but that H^+ was at low levels and below detection on most days. Similarly, a panel study from Birmingham, UK has recently shown no associations with aerosol strong acid in children with and without asthma, during winter and summer monitoring periods, although H^+ levels were very low (Ward *et al.*, 2002). Thus, it appears that when H^+ is present at lower levels, the sulphate association with health effects is weakened, which agrees with biological plausibility that strongly acidic sulphates (such as sulphuric acid and ammonium bisulphate) should be more deleterious to health than more neutralised forms of sulphate (e.g. ammonium sulphate).

More recently, Klemm and Mason (2000), as a part of the Aerosol Research and Inhalation Epidemiology (ARIES) Study, analysed 12 months of PM components data in Atlanta for their associations with daily mortality, reporting no significant sulphate or H^+ associations with daily mortality. They used Poisson generalised linear model adjusting for weather and seasonal cycles. However, the major weakness of the Klemm and Mason analysis of Atlanta data is its short study period. Given the expected effect size of sulphate and other PM mass indices from the literature, and considering the modest population size in Atlanta, one would not expect to be able to detect significant associations between mortality and air pollution, with only one year of data. It is therefore not appropriate to emphasise the lack of statistical significance in these results. Indeed, the reported PM mass and sulphate effect estimates reported, though not statistically significant, are in fact in the range of effect size estimates reported in other studies. Overall, the Klemm and Mason (2000) Atlanta study effect results are not inconsistent with other studies showing $PM_{2.5}$ and sulphate associations with mortality and morbidity, once its statistical limitations are considered.

Thus, while attempts to correlate human mortality with present day ambient acid aerosol concentrations have found mixed results, this appears to be in part explainable by the differing levels of acid aerosol exposure and statistical power across the studies. Clearly, there is a critical need for more such present day acid aerosol studies to be conducted, in order to determine whether the Buffalo results indicating both acute morbidity and mortality effects at ambient H^+ levels can be confirmed at other locales where H^+ is measurable. Equally, data from other parts of the world are also needed to determine the transferability of these North American results.

Studies relating health effects to long-term acid aerosol exposures

A limited but growing amount of epidemiologic study data currently exist by which to evaluate possible relationships between chronic exposures to ambient acid aerosols and human health effects.

Acid mists exposure in Japan

Kitagawa (1984) examined the cause of the Yokkaichi asthma events (1960 to 1969) and concluded that the observed respiratory diseases were not due to sulphur dioxide, but to concentrated sulphuric acid mists emitted from stacks of calciners of a titanium oxide manufacturing plant located windward of the residential area. This was based on the fact that the SO_3/SO_2 ratio of 0.48 was much higher than the normal range of 0.02 to 0.05. The acid particles were fairly large (0.7 to 3.3 um) compared with acid aerosols usually seen in the US, but were still were in the respirable range. Respiratory morbidity prevalence in the vicinity fell markedly after the installation of electrostatic precipitators that reduced H_2SO_4 and other particulate matter emissions.

Studies relating chronic health effects to acid aerosols

In a hypothesis generating discussion, Speizer (1989) utilised pollution data that Spengler *et al.* (1989) gathered in 4 of the 6 cities. It should be noted that these data may contain unaddressed bronchitis variation due to factors other than pollution, so the relationship of bronchitis rates with pollution in these preliminary analyses must be considered as being only suggestive. However, when the city-specific bronchitis rates are plotted against mean H^+ and PM_{15} concentrations, there is a relative shift in the ordering of the cities which suggests a better correlation of bronchitis prevalence with H^+ than with PM_{15} (see Fig. 3).

Damokosh *et al.* (1993) analysed the 6-Cities' paediatric bronchitis data more thoroughly by incorporating controls for confounding variables, and also added a seventh locale, Kanahwa County, WV to the analysis. Respiratory health status was assessed via a parent-completed questionnaire and nine indicators of asthmatic and bronchitic symptom reports were considered. Significant associations were found between summer mean H^+ and bronchitis and related symptoms

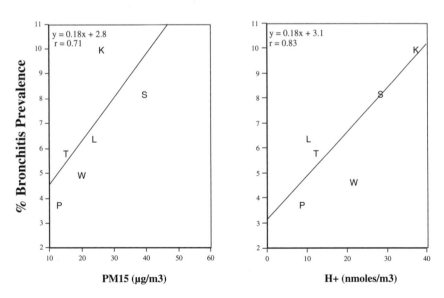

Fig. 3.   Bronchitis in children 10 to 12 years in 6 US Cities (Source: Speizer, 1989; Dockery, 1993).

(cough, phlegm, and chest illness). The estimated relative odds for bronchitic symptoms associated with the lowest mean value of particle strong acidity (15.7 nmoles/m^3) to the highest (57.8 nmoles/m^3) was 2.4 (95% CI: 1.9 to 3.2). No associations were found for asthma or asthma related symptoms (doctor diagnosed asthma, chronic wheeze, and wheeze with attacks of shortness of breath). However, equivalent results were found with other particle mass measurements highly correlated with aerosol acidity.

As a follow-up to the 6-Cities study, the relationship of respiratory symptom/illness reporting with chronic exposures to acidic aerosols (annual mean particulate strong acidity concentrations ranging from 0.5 to 52 nmoles/m^3) was tested among a cohort of schoolchildren in 24 rural and suburban communities in the United States and Canada (Dockery *et al.*, 1996). Questionnaires were completed by the parents of 15,523 schoolchildren aged 8 to 12 years of age. Bronchitic and asthmatic symptoms were considered separately and city-specific reporting rates calculated after adjustment for the effects of gender, age, parental asthma, parental education and parental allergies. Increased reporting of bronchial symptoms were also associated with other measures of particulate air pollution including sulphate — relative odds 1.7 (95% CI: 1.1 to 2.4). While asthmatic symptom reports were not statistically significant with any of the air pollutants, including particulate acidity, bronchitic symptoms were, especially with particulate strong acidity (relative odds 1.7, 95% CI: 1.1 to 2.5) across the range of exposures.

Raizenne *et al.* (1996) used the same cohort of over 10,750 children described above to examine the effects on pulmonary function again employing a patient-completed questionnaire, but with each child performing a standardized forced expiratory maneuver on one occasion between October and May. Air and meteorological monitoring was performed in each community for the year preceding the pulmonary function tests. A two-stage logistic regression analysis was used, adjusting for age, sex, height, weight, sex-height interaction and parental history of asthma. Residence in high particle strong acidity regions was associated on average with a 3.41% (95% CI: 4.72, 2.09) and a 2.95% (95% CI: 4.36, 1.52) lower than predicted FVC and FEV$_1$, respectively for a 52 nmoles/m^3 difference in H$^+$. For children with a measured FVC less than or equal to 85% of predicted, the odds ratio for lower lung function was 2.5 (95% CI: 1.7, 3.6) across the range of H^+ exposures. Assuming that these exposures reflect lifetime exposure of the children in this study, the data suggest that long-term exposure to ambient particle acidity may have a deleterious effect on normal lung growth, development and function.

Cross-sectional epidemiological studies suggest that sulphate-associated fine particles (i.e. fossil fuel combustion products) are among the most toxic. Dockery *et al.* (1993) reported the results of a prospective cohort study in six US cities, in which the effects of air pollution on mortality were estimated, controlling for individual risk factors. Survival analysis, including Cox proportional-hazards regression modelling, was conducted with data from a 14 to 16 year mortality follow-up of 8,111 adults. After adjusting for smoking and other risk factors, statistically significant associations were found between air pollution and mortality. Using inhalable particles, fine particles, or sulphates as the indicator of pollution, they all gave similar results of an adjusted mortality-rate ratio for the most polluted city, as compared with the least polluted city of 1.26 (95% CI = 1.08 to 1.47). Weaker mortality associations were found with H^+ than for other PM metrics (such as SO_4 or $PM_{2.5}$) in this analysis (Fig. 4), although the data were again limited by missing H^+ data. Also, while other pollutants' data collection spanned the study period of this multi-year study, H^+ data were only collected for a short period (usually less than one year) near the end of this study, and this was used to characterise lifetime exposures of adult study participants. This seems especially inappropriate in Steubenville, OH, where the industrial (i.e. steel mill) pollution levels declined during the course of the study, as the steel industry in the valley declined. Moreover, as shown in Fig. 5, different times of the year were sampled in each city, which affects the inter-city comparisons, since H^+ is considerably higher in summer than winter in the US. In some cities such as Harriman, sampling focused more on the high H^+ summer period, while in Steubenville, OH, the H^+ data were also collected through two low H^+ winters, resulting in a much lower mean. Note also that different years were sampled in different cities, as the H^+ sampling equipment was "cycled" through the 6 cities. In light of these city-to city differences in H^+ sampling period,

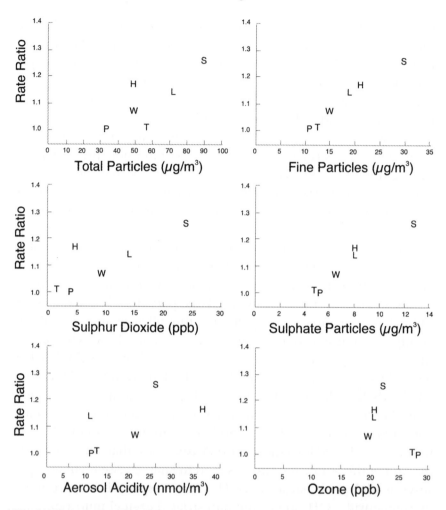

Fig. 4. Estimated adjusted mortality-rate ratios and pollution levels in the six cities (Dockery *et al.*, 1993).

it is perhaps not surprising that Steubenville had the lowest $H^+/SO_4^=$ ratio. In contrast, the inhalable particle, fine particle, and sulphate data employed in each city were much more representative, having been collected earlier and approximately over a five-to six-year period in these cities. These issues, along with others, perhaps explain why this study was unable to find a statistically significant correlation

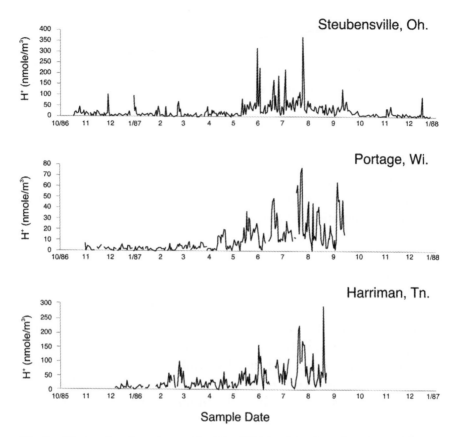

Fig. 5. Time-series plots of aerosol acidity (H$^+$) levels in three "six city study" cities (Spengler *et al.*, 1990).

between H$^+$ and mortality (relative to sulphates and fine particles, for example) as, in a large part, the H$^+$ data employed were apparently not appropriate for this application.

Although it considered sulphates and not H$^+$ directly, a recent study extending follow-up analysis of the ACS data (Pope, 2000) has confirmed the original associations of long-term sulphates and PM$_{2.5}$ exposures with human cardiovascular mortality. This study also found cancer deaths to be associated with sulphate-containing aerosols. The cancer risk of living in a polluted US city was comparable to that from living with a smoker.

Summary of epidemiology evidence

Historical and present-day epidemiological evidence suggest that there can be both acute and chronic human health effects associated with exposure to ambient atmospheres containing strongly acidic PM. Evidence from historical pollution for episodes, notably the London Fog episodes of the 1950s and early 1960s, indicate that extremely elevated daily acid aerosol concentrations (of the order of $400\,\mu g/m^3$ as H_2SO_4, or roughly $8{,}000\,nmoles/m^3$ H^+) may be associated with excess mortality when present as a co-pollutant with elevated concentrations of Black Smoke (BS) and SO_2 an effect also present in non-episode situations where acid levels were lower ($\leq 30\,\mu g/m^3$ as H_2SO_4, or $\leq$ approximately $600\,nmoles/m^3$ H^+). Two attempts to relate present-day levels of acidic aerosols with acute and chronic mortality in the USA were unable to do so, but there may not have been a sufficiently large enough set of H^+ data to detect H^+ and health associations in these studies. The 6-Cities dataset, also showed weaker associations between H^+ and daily mortality than with fine particles and sulphates, although the H^+ dataset was much less robust than that for the other PM metrics, while a much more extensive two-and-a-half year record of daily H^+ measurements in Buffalo, NY, revealed H^+ to be among one of them most consistently associated with adverse morbidity and mortality.

Associations between ambient acidic aerosols and summertime respiratory hospital admissions in North America have been demonstrated in the recent past, significant independent H^+ effects remaining even after simultaneously considering the other major co-pollutant, O_3, in the regression model. In the Toronto analysis, the increase in respiratory hospital admissions associated with H^+ was approximately six times that of non-acidic PM_{10} (per unit mass). In these studies, H^+ effects were estimated to be the largest during acid aerosol episodes ($H^+ \geq 10\,\mu g/m^3$ as H_2SO_4, or $\sim 200\,nmoles/m^3$ H^+), which occur ~ 2 to 3 times per year in Eastern North America. These studies suggest that present-day strongly acidic aerosols may represent a portion of PM that is associated with acute respiratory health effects in the general population in North America, although similar data are not available for other parts of the world.

Studies of the effects of chronic H^+ exposures on children's respiratory health and lung function reveal bronchitis prevalence rates in the 6-Cities to be more closely associated with average H^+ concentrations than with PM in general, with a relative odds of bronchitic symptoms of about two and a half for the highest versus the lowest acid concentration. This is supported by a follow-up study of children in 24 US and Canadian communities, where bronchitic symptoms were significantly associated with strongly acidic PM (relative odds = 1.7). It was also found in the 24-Cities study that mean FVC and FEV_1 were lower in locales having high particle strong acidity. However, one study of children in the urban Midlands of the UK showed no such associations. Thus, chronic exposure to strongly acidic PM may have effects on measures of respiratory health in children, at least in North America.

6. Toxicological Evidence

Given the indications of an association between exposure to ambient acidic aerosols and health effects from the results of epidemiological studies, there has been much interest in evaluating the "biological plausibility" for such an association. To this end, this section reviews the toxicology of acid sulphate particles based on controlled exposure studies in animals and in humans. Unfortunately, most of the available tocicological data have been derived primarily using pure aerosols of ammonium sulphate [$(NH_4)_2SO_4$], ammonium bisulphate (NH_4HSO_4), or sulphuric acid (H_2SO_4), which limits those results' applicability to real-world situations, in which acidic sulphate aerosols are usually formed heterogeneously on pre-existing ambient particles. Fortunately, some studies have been done looking at interactions between acidity and combustion particles (e.g. residual oil fly ash, ROFA), and these studies provide information that is possibly more relevant to real-world acidic PM exposures.

Mortality

High exposure concentrations of sulphuric acid, generally above $4 \, mg/m^3$, are needed for lethality in animals, while lethal concentrations for other acid sulphates are higher still. Commonly seen pulmonary lesions include focal atelectasis, hemorrhage, congestion, pulmonary and perivascular edema, and epithelial desquamation of bronchioles; hyperinflation is also often evident.

Pulmonary mechanical function

Controlled clinical studies of healthy adults have shown no consistent significant effects on pulmonary function nor respiratory symptoms with acute exposure to H_2SO_4 at concentrations $\leq 1 \, mg/m^3$ (0.1–1 μm diameter), even with exercise (Avol *et al.*, 1988; Frampton, *et al.*, 1992; U. S. Environmental Protection Agency, 1989; Tunnicliffe *et al.*, 2001), although there are some suggestions that doses such as these potentiate the effects of allergen responsiveness in asthmatics (Tunnicliffe *et al.*, 2001). Acute exposures at higher concentrations using larger particles, in the 10–20 μm range characteristic of those which may occur in acidic fogs, have been associated with some increased respiratory symptoms, e.g. cough, but without any effects on lung function parameters (Avol *et al.*, 1988; Linn *et al.*, 1989). On the other hand, there is some evidence that asthmatics may be more sensitive than healthy individuals to the effects on lung mechanical function and that they may experience modest bronchoconstriction following exposure to H_2SO_4 at concentrations $< 1 \, mg/m^3$ (Avol *et al.*, 1988; Tunnicliffe *et al.*, 2001; Avol *et al.*, 1998; Linn *et al.*, 1989; Koenig *et al.*, 1993).

All asthmatics may not be equally sensitive to acid sulphates. While elderly asthmatics do not appear to be a susceptible population (Koenig *et al.*, 1993), adolescents with allergic asthma do. Small declines in FEV_1 were noted only after a 40 min exposure to H_2SO_4 (0.6 μm) at $0.068 \, mg/m^3$ in one study (Koenig *et al.*, 1983), although effects on lung function have not been consistently observed at exposure concentrations $< 0.1 \, mg/m^3$ (Koenig *et al.*, 1992). It is likely that the specific characteristics of the asthmatic population studied plays a significant role in sensitivity to acid exposure and the resultant effective concentration.

The effects of acid sulphates on healthy humans are consistent with those observed in experimental toxicology assessments, in that acute exposures of most species of healthy animals at H_2SO_4 concentrations $\leq 1 \, mg/m^3$ ($< 1 \, \mu m$ diameter) have not been shown to alter standard lung function tests (U. S. Environmental Protection Agency, 1989). The notable exception is the guinea pig, which appears to be especially sensitive and shows pulmonary functional changes at H_2SO_4 levels well below $1 \, mg/m^3$. Perhaps the guinea pig may be a model of a susceptible human population, since these animals actually show a dyspneic response following sulphur oxide exposure that is quite similar to asthma episodes in humans, in terms of the rapidity of onset and associated obstructive pulmonary functional changes.

While lung function generally will not be affected in normal animals and humans by acid sulphate exposure, an increase in airway reactivity was observed with broncho-constrictor challenge, following exposure to $1 \, mg/m^3$ H_2SO_4 for 16 minutes, and in some adult asthmatics, following exposure to $0.1 \, mg/m^3$ (Utell *et al.*, 1983), which coheres on the UK work on potentiation of allergen response by $1mg/m^3$ H_2SO_4 (Tunnicliffe *et al.*, 2001). There was also some indication of a delayed response, following exposure in the former study. However, there appears to be no consistent effect of acute exposure to H_2SO_4 on airway reactivity in healthy or asthmatic individuals, in that other studies have failed to show alterations in reactivity at concentrations up to $2 \, mg/m^3$, with either acid fog droplets or sub-micrometer acid particles (Avol *et al.*, 1988; Avol *et al.*, 1988; Linn *et al.*, 1989).

The ability of H_2SO_4 to alter airway responsiveness has been assessed in a number of studies using various animals. While acute exposures of healthy guinea pigs have shown inconsistent results, with effective concentrations ranging from $0.2 \, mg/m^3$ to $> 1 \, mg/m^3$ (Kobayashi and Shinozaki 1993; Silbaugh *et al.*, 1981), chronic exposures of healthy rabbits to $0.25 \, mg/m^3$ ($0.3 \, \mu m$; $1 \, h/d$, $5 \, d/wk$ for $4 \, mo$) induced nonspecific airway hyper-responsiveness (Gearhart and Schlesinger, 1986). Furthermore, a single exposure of rabbits to $0.075 \, mg/m^3$ H_2SO_4 was also shown to induce nonspecific hyper-responsiveness, using an *in vitro* airway preparation (el-Fawal and Schlesinger, 1994).

Thus, while controlled exposures to acid sulphates have produced transient changes in pulmonary function in asthmatics, including enhanced nonspecific airway hyper-responsiveness in some cases, and epidemiological evidence indicates that exacerbation of symptoms in asthmatics may be related to atmospheric particulate acids, the contribution of chronic ambient sulphur oxide exposure to the development of airway dysfunction in normal individuals remains unclear.

Pulmonary defenses

Acidic sulphates can affect various aspects of pulmonary defenses, such as mucociliary transport, alveolar clearance of deposited particles, and pulmonary macrophage function. Acute exposure to H_2SO_4 at levels as low as $0.1\,mg/m^3$ (0.3–$0.6\,\mu m$ diameter) alters mucociliary transport in healthy humans (Leikauf *et al.*, 1981; Spektor *et al.*, 1989); any special sensitivity of mucociliary transport in asthmatics has not been demonstrated (Spektor *et al.*, 1985; Laube *et al.*, 1993). Furthermore, such exposures result in qualitatively similar effects on mucociliary clearance in humans and various animal species, in that the nature of clearance change, i.e. slowing or speeding, is exposure-concentration-dependent, with stimulation of clearance occurring at low concentrations and retardation at higher levels (Schlesinger, 1990). Furthermore, partially or totally neutralized sulphates are less effective than sulphuric acid in altering clearance function (Schlesinger, 1984). Chronic exposure to sulphur oxides may also affect tracheo-bronchial mucociliary clearance. Rabbits exposed to H_2SO_4 at 0.125–$0.25\,mg/m^3$ ($0.3\,\mu m$ diameter; $1, 2\,h/d$, $5\,d/wk$) showed acceleration or retardation of clearance rate, depending on the concentration (Schlesinger, 1990).

Clearance of particles from the alveolar region is also affected by acidic sulphates. Exposure to H_2SO_4 results in either accelerated or retarded particle clearance from the alveolar region, depending on the exposure regime and animal species examined, and the effective concentrations range from $0.25\,mg/m^3$ (Schlesinger, 1990; Phalen *et al.*, 1980). As with other biological endpoints, the partially or totally neutralized sulphates are less effective in this regard (Schlesinger, 1989).

The alveolar macrophage is important in clearance function, as well as other aspects of lung defense. At levels $\leq 1\,mg/m^3$, sulphuric acid affects certain functions of macrophages lavaged from various species, following single or repeated inhalation exposure. This includes phagocytic activity, adherence, random mobility, intracellular pH and the release or production of certain cytokines (e.g. TNFα and IL1β and reactive oxygen species (Schlesinger, 1990; Zelikoff *et al.*, 1994; Zelikoff and Schlesinger, 1992; Chen *et al.*, 1995). Such effects may ultimately be reflected in an altered ability of these cells to adequately perform their role in host defenses, including particle clearance and anti-microbial activity. However, the evidence that sulphuric acid reduces resistance to bacterial infection is conflicting, and may depend on the animal model used (U. S. Environmental Protection Agency, 1989; Zelikoff and Schlesinger, 1992).

Most of the database involving effects of sulphur oxides on lung defense is concerned with non-specific, i.e. non-immunologic, mechanisms. The little available evidence on pulmonary humoral or cell-mediated immunity provides only equivocal indication of the ability of sulphur oxides to enhance sensitisation to antigens (Osebold *et al.*, 1980) or to modulate the activity of cells involved in allergic responses (Riedel *et al.*, 1988; Fujimaki *et al.*, 1992).

Pulmonary morphology and biochemistry

Acute or chronic exposures to H_2SO_4 at high levels ($\gg 1 \, mg/m^3$) are associated with a number of characteristic responses in animals, e.g. alveolitis, bronchial and/or bronchiolar epithelial desquamation, and edema (Brownstein, 1980; Schwartz *et al.*, 1977). However, the sensitivity of morphologic endpoints is dependent on the animal species, with the rat being apparently the least sensitive and the guinea pig being the most sensitive (Schwartz *et al.*, 1977; Wolff, 1986; Cavender *et al.*, 1977). In many cases, the nature of lesions in different species are similar, but differed in location. This is perhaps a reflection of interspecies differences in the deposition pattern of the acid particles.

Acute exposure to H_2SO_4 at $\leq 1 \, mg/m^3$ does not produce evidence of inflammatory responses in humans or animals (Frampton *et al.*, 1992; U. S. Environmental Protection Agency, 1989). Although one study indicated a change in airway permeability with exposure of guinea pigs to $0.3 \, mg/m^3$ ($3 \, h/d$, 1 or $4 \, d$) (Chen *et al.*, 1992), most others using concentrations $\geq 1 \, mg/m^3$ reported no such effects (Wolff *et al.*, 1986; Warren and Last, 1987). Chronic exposures to

$\leq 1\,\mathrm{mg/m^3}$ produce a response characterised by alterations in the epithelial secretory cells. For example, rabbits exposed to 0.125–0.5 mg/m³ H_2SO_4 (0.3 µm diameter) for 1, 2 h/d, 5 d/wk (Gearhart and Schlesinger, 1988; Schlesinger et al., 1992) showed increases in the relative number density of bronchial secretory cells extending to the bronchiolar level. These changes began within 4 weeks of exposures, and persisted till 3 mo following the end of exposure.

Toxicology of acidic PM in compromised host animal models

Some epidemiological studies suggest that there may be sub-groups of the population that may be especially susceptible to effects from inhaled particles, particularly those with lung diseases. However, most toxicology studies have used healthy adult animals, and there are very few data to allow examination of the effects of different disease states on the biological response to PM. Alterations in deposition sites and clearance rates and pathways by concurrent disease may impact upon dose delivered from inhaled particles and ultimate toxicity, but this has not been studied in detail.

Mechanisms of toxicity due to the inhalation of pure acidic aerosols

The exact mechanisms underlying the toxicity of acidic particles or vapors to the respiratory tract are not known with certainty. The responses to acidic sulphate particles likely result from the deposition of H^+ on airway surfaces (U.S. Environmental Protection Agency, 1989; Zelikoff et al., 1994; Schlesinger and Chen, 1994). Examination of diverse biological endpoints has shown that the relative potency of acidic sulphate aerosols is related to their degree of acidity, i.e. the H^+ content within the exposure environment (Koenig et al., 1993; Schlesinger, 1984; Zelikoff et al., 1994; Schlesinger et al., 1990). However, as to which metric for H^+ concentration better relates to these responses, i.e. whether it is total available H^+ concentration measured as titratable acidity in lung fluids following deposition, or free H^+ concentration, measured by pH (Fine et al., 1987), remains unclear.

Since the hydrogen ion is likely to be responsible for the toxicity of acid sulphates, the mode of inhalation will affect the potential for biological response. For the same mass (ionic) concentration of acidic sulphates in an exposure atmosphere, oral inhalation will result in more neutralisation, compared with nasal inhalation, and therefore, less H^+ available for deposition within the lower respiratory tract (Larson *et al.*, 1982). The extent of neutralisation of inhaled acid sulphates has in fact been shown to modulate toxic effects. Asthmatic subjects inhaling H_2SO_4 demonstrated greater responses when exposure was conducted under conditions in which oral ammonia levels were low, compared with when they were high (Utell *et al.*, 1989).

If the responses to deposited acidic sulphate particles involve local changes in pH at sites at which these particles land (Last *et al.*, 1984; Hattis *et al.*, 1987), then a critical number of such particles must be deposited at such sites in order to deliver sufficient H^+ so as to alter local pH. It has been demonstrated that the number of particles within an exposure atmosphere, rather than just the total mass concentration of H^+, is an important factor in determining whether any response follows inhalation of acidic sulphates (Chen *et al.*, 1995) and that there is a threshold for both number concentration and mass concentration.

Sulphuric acid is a broncho-active agent that can produce constriction of smooth muscle. This results from irritant receptor stimulation following direct contact by deposited acid particles, and/or from humoral mediators such as histamine, released as a result of exposure (Charles and Menzel, 1975). Furthermore, since hypo-osmolar aerosols can induce broncho-constriction in some asthmatics and acidity may potentiate broncho-constriction caused by hypo-osmolar particles (Balmes *et al.*, 1988), the molarity of inhaled acid sulphate particles may be a factor in eliciting responses in susceptible individuals.

Acid sulphate-induced airway hyper-responsiveness may involve an increased sensitivity to mediators involved in the control of airway smooth muscle tone. Guinea pigs exposed to H_2SO_4 showed a small degree of enhanced response to histamine, but a much more pronounced sensitivity to substance P, a neuropeptide with effects on bronchial smooth muscle (Stengel *et al.*, 1993). Inhalation of H_2SO_4 has also been shown to upset the balance of eicosanoid synthesis/metabolism, which is necessary for the maintenance of pulmonary homeostasis (Schlesinger *et al.*, 1990). Since some eicosanoids are involved in the regulation of smooth muscle tone, this imbalance may also be involved in the development of airway hyper-responsiveness. For example, incubation of rabbit tracheal explants in acidic media reduced the production of prostaglandin E2 (Schlesinger *et al.*, 1990), an epithelial-derived mediator associated with bronchodilation and the inhibition of agonist-induced smooth muscle contraction.

Modulation of pulmonary pharmacological receptors may underlie some sulphur oxide-induced responses. In terms of airway hyperresponsiveness, this could involve interference with normal contractile/dilatory processes in the airways, via modulation of receptors involved in the maintenance of muscle tone (el-Fawal and Schlesinger, 1994).

β-adrenergic stimulation down-regulates pulmonary macrophage function, and this has been shown to be influenced by short term, repeated exposures of rabbits to H_2SO_4 (McGovern, 1993). Any acid-induced enhanced down-regulation, by affecting production of reactive oxygen species by macrophages, may create an environment conducive for secondary pulmonary insult such as bacterial infections, especially in susceptible populations. In addition, alterations in the mediator release from the macrophage due to receptor down regulation, may in turn influence airway responsiveness.

Finally, one of the mechanisms underlying acid sulphate-induced exacerbation of asthmatic symptoms may be increased airway epithelial permeability, with subsequent enhanced penetration of inhaled antigens, present in most ambient atmospheres, to submucosal cells involved in allergic reactions.

A perviously noted, acidic particles which deposit upon airway surfaces can be buffered in airway fluids. However, the buffering capacity of mucus may be altered in individuals with compromised lungs. For example, sputum (which contains mucus and other fluids) from asthmatics was found to have a reduced buffering capacity compared with that from normals (Holma, 1985), and this may at least in part underlie some of their sensitivity to acidic sulphates.

One of the most studied responses to acid sulphates is the change in tracheobronchial mucociliary transport. High exposure concentrations of H_2SO_4 are needed to affect ciliary beating (Schiff *et al.*, 1979; Grose *et al.*, 1980), so any effects, especially at lower levels, are likely to be due to changes in the mucus lining itself, such as a change in its rheological properties. At alkaline pH, mucus is more fluid than at acidic pH, so a small increase in viscosity due to deposited acid, could "stiffen" the mucus blanket, altering the efficiency with which it is coupled to the beating cilia (Knorst *et al.*, 1994; Holma *et al.*, 1977).

Another mechanism by which acidic sulphates may affect mucociliary clearance is via alteration in the rate and/or amount of mucus secreted. A small increase in mucus production could facilitate clearance, while more excessive production could result in a thickened mucus layer which would be ineffectively coupled to the cilia. Chronic exposure of animals to sulphuric acid has been shown to increase the number of airway secretory cells, especially in small airways where these cells are normally absent or few in number (Gearhart and Schlesinger, 1988). Furthermore, this increase has been associated with a change in the glycoprotein composition of the mucus, suggesting increased viscosity. The result of any increase in cells could be an increase in secretory rate or volume. While mucus hyper-secretion is a hallmark of chronic bronchitis, epidemiological studies are not clear as to its importance in the development of chronic pulmonary diseases related to air pollution (Peto *et al.*, 1983).

The airways actively transport ions and the interaction between trans-epithelial ion transport and consequent fluid movement is important in the maintenance of the mucus lining. A change in ion transport due to deposited acid particles may alter the depth and/or composition of the sol layer of the mucus blanket (Nathanson and Nadel, 1984), perhaps affecting clearance rate.

An effect of acidic sulphate exposure, which may be related to a number of physiological alterations, involves changes in cellular pH. Intracellular pH is one of the major determinants of the rate of many cellular functions and has been linked to the control of vital cellular processes. Alveolar macrophages obtained from guinea pigs exposed to H_2SO_4 showed alterations in internal pH regulation, which was attributable to effects on the Na^+/H^+ exchanger located within the cell membrane (Qu *et al.*, 1993). Deposited acid may also affect the internal pH of epithelial cells and other functions of these cells.

One of the more controversial biological responses to sulphuric acid is the development of cancer. Various potential mechanisms may underlie any link to carcinogenesis, such as pH modulation of other xenobiotics or low pH-induced changes in cells, in terms of mitotic and enzyme regulation (Cookfair *et al.*, 1985). However, the most likely being irritation, the result of acid-induced chronic inflammation, culminating in increased cell proliferation, as suggested by the finding of an increased incidence of laryngeal cancer in a study involving sulphuric acid exposed workers (Coggon *et al.*, 1996). The ability of sulphuric acid to act as a tumor promoter was suggested by a study in rats chronically exposed to sulphuric acid and nitrogen dioxide (Ichinose and Sagai, 1992). Clearly, the issue of sulphuric acid carcinogenicity is not resolved.

Toxicology of mixtures containing acids

Although human contact with ambient air pollution usually involves simultaneous exposure to more than one chemical, and biological responses to the inhalation of polluted atmospheres may depend on the interplay between individual chemicals, experimental studies have routinely examined effects resulting from single pollutants. As a result, public health standards have generally been set without regard for potential interactions between the materials being regulated. However, characterisation of effects from exposures to relevant mixtures of air pollutants is necessary for appropriate assessment of health risks in the real world.

Most toxicologic studies of pollutant mixtures involved exposures to mixtures containing only two materials, given either simultaneously or sequentially. A number of controlled exposure studies have indicated that significant toxicological interactions may occur between acid sulphates and other pollutants, the most notable of which is ozone (Linn *et al.*, 1994; Schlesinger *et al.*, 1992). However, the nature or extent of interaction appears to depend on the exposure regimen, biological endpoints and animal species used, and no unifying principles or consistent conclusions are evident (Schlesinger, 1995; Amdur *et al.*, 1986).

A few studies have examined the effects of exposure to multicomponent atmospheres containing acidic sulphate particles. No change in particle clearance from the tracheobronchial tree or respiratory region was seen after a 4-hour exposure of rats to a SO_2-sulphate mix, consisting of SO_2 (5 ppm) plus $1.5 \, mg/m^3$ ($0.5 \, \mu m$, MMAD) of an aerosol containing $(NH_4)_2SO_4$ and $Fe_2(SO_4)_3$ (Mannix *et al.*, 1982). Mice exposed (5 hour/d, 5 d/week for 103 d) to mixtures of O_3 (0.1 ppm), SO_2 (5 ppm) and $(NH_4)_2SO_4$ ($1.04 \, mg/m^3$) showed enhanced bactericidal activity of macrophages, compared with O_3 alone (Aranyi *et al.*, 1983). This same exposure regime also resulted in a greater (compared to O_3 alone) degree of *in vitro* cytostasis to tumour target cells co-cultured with peritoneal macrophages obtained from exposed mice.

Kleinman *et al.* (1985) exposed rats for 4 hours to atmospheres consisting of various combinations of O_3 (0.6 ppm), NO_2 (2.5 ppm), SO_2 (5 ppm) and particles. The latter consisted of $1 \, mg/m^3$ ($0.2 \, \mu m$, MMAD) of either $(NH_4)_2SO_4$ or H_2SO_4, laced with iron and manganese sulphates. The metallic salts acted as catalysts for the conversion of sulphur [IV] into sulphur [VI], and the incorporation of gases into the aerosol droplets. A significant enhancement of tissue damage was produced by exposure to atmospheres containing H_2SO_4 (or HNO_3), compared with those containing $(NH_4)_2SO_4$. In addition, there was a suggestion that the former atmospheres resulted in a greater area of the lung developing a thickening of the alveolar walls, cellular infiltration into the interstitium and an increase in free cells within the alveolar spaces.

To assess the effects of acid exposure on macrophage function, rats were exposed to pollutant mixtures (0.3 ppm O_3, 1.2 ppm NO_2, 2.5 ppm SO_2, $270 \, \mu g/m^3$ $(NH_4)_2SO_4$, $220 \, \mu g/m^3$ $Fe_2(SO_4)_3$ and $4 \, \mu g/m^3$ $MnSO_4$) for 4 hour/d for 7 or 21 days (Prasad *et al.*, 1988). The activity of macrophage surface receptors (Fc) was reduced to a greater extent after 21 d of exposure than after 7 d; in both cases, the reduction persisting for up to 3 d post-exposure. Macrophage phagocytic activity was reduced after 7 d of exposure, but not after 21 d. Similar findings were found for exposure to $0.46 \, mg/m^3$ diesel exhaust particles ($0.15 \, \mu m$), $400 \, \mu g/m^3$ HNO_3 vapor, and $180 \, \mu g/m^2$ H_2SO_4 (present as a surface coat on the diesel particles). In both sets of experiments, interaction could not be determined, since the individual components were not tested separately.

In a later study, the same group (Prasad *et al.*, 1990) examined particle clearance, lung histology and macrophage phagocytic activity following nose-only exposures of rats (Sprague-Dawley, M, 6 week) for 5 hour/d for 5 d to atmospheres consisting of 0.39 mg/m^3 HNO$_3$ vapor, 0.55 mg/m^3 diesel exhaust particles, and 0.19 mg/m^3 sulphuric acid coated on the diesel particles. There was no change in tracheobronchial or alveolar clearance of tracer particles with this mixture, compared with air controls. While no deep lung lesions nor any change in the turnover rate of the epithelial cells from the nose, trachea or alveolar region were noted, there was a decrease in the percentage of macrophages which had internalised diesel particles following exposure to the mixture, compared with cells recovered from animals exposed to the diesel particles alone. Furthermore, phagocytosis was depressed up to 3 d following exposure to the mixture.

Amdur and Chen (1989) exposed guinea pigs to simulated primary emissions from coal combustion processes, produced by mixing ZnO, sulphur dioxide and water in a high temperature combustion furnace. The animals were exposed for 3 hour/d for 5 d to ultrafine (0.05 μm CMD, σg = 2) aerosols of zinc oxide (ZnO) having a surface coating of H$_2$SO$_4$ resulting from this process. Levels of sulphur dioxide ranged from 0.2–1 ppm. Acid sulphate concentrations as low as 0.02–0.03 mg/m^3, as equivalent H$_2$SO$_4$, delivered in this manner resulted in significant reductions in total lung volume, vital capacity and DLco. The effects appeared to be cumulative, in that their severity increased with increasing exposure duration. Increases in the protein content of pulmonary lavage fluid, as well as an increase in PMNs, were seen but much higher exposure levels of pure H$_2$SO$_4$ aerosol were needed to produce comparable results, suggesting that the physical state of the associated acid in a pollutant mixture is an important determinant of response. However, a confounder in these studies is that the number concentration was greater for the coated particles than the pure acid particles.

Other studies have examined responses to acid-coated particles. Chen *et al.* (1989) exposed (nose-only) guinea pigs (male, Hartley, 250–300 g) for 3 hours to ultrafine ZnO (0.05 μm, σg = 1.86) layered with 0.025 or 0.084 mg/m^3 H$_2$SO$_4$. Immediately following exposure, animals exposed to the higher acid concentration showed increased levels of prostaglandin F2α, compared with those found in animals exposed to ZnO alone. Levels of prostaglandins E1 and 6-keto-PGF1α, thromboxane B_2 and leukotriene B_4 were similar to those found in animals exposed to the metal alone. During the post-exposure period, changes in prostaglandin E_1, leukotriene B_4 and thromboxane B_2 were noted.

Guinea pigs exposed to acid coated ZnO for 1 hour (equivalent concentrations of H_2SO_4 of 0.020 and 0.030 mg/m^3 n the 0.05 μm ZnO particles), and to pure H_2SO_4 droplets showed hyperresponsiveness in animals exposed to the acid-coated particles, but not in those exposed to furnace gases (control) or to the metal oxide alone (Chen *et al.*, 1992). A similar quantitative change was noted in those animals exposed to the pure droplet at $\sim 10x$ the concentration of the coated particles (Amdur and Chen, 1989), suggesting that the exposure to particles under conditions that promote the formation of acid as a surface coating on respirable particles can induce nonspecific airway hyper-responsiveness. Furthermore, in this case, the size of both the coated and pure acid was the same, suggesting that the coated particles themselves were more effective in eliciting a response than the pure acid.

Effects at similar doses are also seen in gas transfer, both with single and multiple doses (Amdur *et al.*, 1986), with evidence for interaction between ozone and acid layered zinc oxide particles, both with respect to gas transfer and lung volumes (Chen *et al.*, 1991).

Acidic particles, transition metals, and oxidative stress

Ambient acid aerosols may also interact with other constituents of the complex particulate mix in ambient air. For example, some studies suggest that the presence of acidity in particles increases the toxicity of PM (e.g. Chen *et al.*, 1990), especially those containing certain metals. Transition metals (e.g. iron and vanadium) can mediate electron transfer via Fenton reactions, causing oxidative stress that leads to cellular damage and have been shown to cause oxidative stress in lung cells (Dreher *et al.*, 1997; Lay *et al.*, 1999), especially in the presence of acid, which increases the solubility of toxic metals, thereby making these metals even more bioavailable. This may be an important pathway by which acidic particles could enhance toxicity of ambient particles, and provide plausible physiological mechanism for the epidemiological findings.

7. Assessment of Health Risk from Ambient Acidic Particles

The database for health impact from exposure to ambient acidic particles, summarised in this chapter, has made it possible to frame a number of issues in a coherent and focused manner. These involve addressing the apparent discrepancies between results from epidemiological studies of ambient acidic aerosols versus controlled exposure studies of pure acidic aerosols.

One key issue is the role of the sulphate ion, and why it generally correlates with mortality, and morbidity as well as, or better than, other metrics of PM pollution. It is extremely unlikely that $SO_4^=$, per se, is a causal factor for adverse health effects. Thus, if it is not, then it must be acting as a surrogate index for one or more other components or chemical interactions occurring in the PM mixture. One possibility in this regard is that the effects are really due to the $PM_{2.5}$ mass, irrespective of particle composition, and that $SO_4^=$ mass concentration is a more stable measurement of airborne $PM_{2.5}$ than is the reported total $PM_{2.5}$ concentration itself. Ambient $PM_{2.5}$ also includes nitrates (primarily ammonium nitrate) and organics formed by photochemical reactions in the atmosphere. There can be considerable volatilisation of these species on sampling filters, resulting in negative mass weighing artifacts, whose magnitude can vary with source strengths and ambient temperature.

Another possibility is that $SO_4^=$ is serving as a surrogate for H^+ and its actions on the particles upon which it condenses upon formation. Some support for this hypothesis is summarised in Tables 3, 4 and 5. The utility of $SO_4^=$ as a surrogate for H^+, especially for time-series studies in a given region without complex topography, is illustrated in Fig. 6, which demonstrates that both H^+ and $SO_4^=$ concentrations are almost the same at two sites that are 60 miles apart, and that the concentration of both ions rise and fall together.

It is also possible that the causal factor in health effects related to acid aerosols exposure is the number concentration, rather than mass concentration, of irritating particles, which would be dominated by

Table 3. Summary of recent epidemiologic study findings.

Associations Between Ambient Air Particulate Matter and Morbidity Indices

General Population

Population	Pollutants Monitored	Effects Reported	Associated Pollutant(s)*	Reference
Metropolitan Toronto Summers 1986–1988	TSP, PM_{10}, $PM_{2.5}$, $SO_4^=$, H^+, O_3	Increased hospital admissions for respiratory diseases	O_3, H^+, $SO_4^=$	Thurston et al. (1994) *Environ Res* **65**:271–290
New York State: Buffalo, Albany Bronx, Westchester Year-round 1988–1990	$SO_4^=$, H^+, O_3	Increased hospital admissions for respiratory diseases in Buffalo and Bronx	O_3, H^+, $SO_4^=$	Thurston et al. (1992) *JEAEE* **2**:429–450
Detroit Summers 1986–1989	PM_{10}, O_3	Increased hospital admissions for respiratory diseases	PM_{10}, O_3	Schwartz (1994) *Am J Crit Care Med* **150**:648–655
Ontario Summers 1983–1988	$SO_4^=$, O_3	Increased hospital admissions for respiratory diseases	O_3, $SO_4^=$	Burnett et al. (1994) *Environ Res* **65**:172–194
Montreal Summers 1984–1988	PM_{10}, $SO_4^=$, O_3	Increased hospital admissions for respiratory diseases	PM_{10}, $SO_4^=$	Delfino et al. (1994) *Environ Res* **67**:1–19

*Associations with $p \leq 0.05$. **Boldface indicates pollutants most highly associated with the effects.**

Table 4. Summary of recent epidemiologic study findings.

Associations Between Ambient Air Particulate Matter and Morbidity and Lung Function Indices

Population	Pollutants Monitored	Children		Reference
		Effects Reported	Associated Pollutant(s)*	
Asymptomatic and symptomatic children Uniontown, PA Summer 1990	PM_{10}, $PM_{2.5}$, $SO_4^=$, H^+, O_3, SO_2	Reduced PEF Symptoms	**H^+**, $SO_4^=$, O_3 **H^+**, $PM_{2.5}$, $SO_4^=$, SO_2, O_3	Neas et al. (1995) Am J Epid **141**:111–122
Asymptomatic and symptomatic children Austrian Alps Summer 1991	PM_{10}, $SO_4^=$, H^+, NH_4^+, O_3, Pollen	Reduced FVC and FEV1 Increased medication usage	**H^+**, **PM_{10}** (not specified)	Studnicka et al. (1995) Am J Respir Crit Care Med **151**:423–430
Asthmatic children Conn. River Valley Summers 1991–1993	$SO_4^=$, H^+, O_3, Pollen	Increased medication usage Symptoms Reduced PEF	O_3, H^+, $SO_4^=$ O_3, H^+, $SO_4^=$ O_3, H^+, $SO_4^=$	Thurston et al. (1994) Presented at 1994 Joint ISEA-ISEE Conf
Children in 7 U.S. cities Yearlong 1985–1988	PM_{10}, $PM_{2.5}$, $SO_4^=$, H^+, O_3, SO_2, NO_2	Increased symptoms of bronchitis	H^+, **$SO_4^=$**, **$PM_{2.5}$**, PM_{10}	Damokosh (1993) ARRD **147**(4):A632
Children in 24 North American cities Year-round 1988–1990	PM_{10}, $PM_{2.1}$, $SO_4^=$, H^+, O_3, SO_2, NO_2	Increased symptoms of bronchitis Decreased FVC and FEV1	H^+, **$SO_4^=$**, **$PM_{2.1}$**, PM_{10} H^+, **$SO_4^=$**, **$PM_{2.1}$**, PM_{10}	Dockery et al. (1993) ARRD **147**(4):A633 Raizenne et al. (1993) ARRD **147**(4):A635
Children in 10 rural Canadian Communities Year-round 1985–1986	PM_{10}, $SO_4^=$, O_3, NO_2, SO_2	Decreased FVC and FEV1	**$SO_4^=$**, O_3	Stern et al. (1994) Environ Res **66**:125–142

*Associations with $p \le 0.05$. **Boldface indicates pollutants most highly associated with the effects.**

Table 5. Components of ambient air particulate matter (PM) that may account for some or all of the effects associated with PM exposures.

Component	Evidence for Role in Effects	Doubts
Strong Acid (H^+)	• Statistical associations with health effects in most recent studies for which ambient H^+ concentrations were measured. • Coherent responses for some health endpoints in human and animal inhalation and *in vitro* studies at environmentally relevant doses.	• Similar PM-associated effects observed in locations with low ambient H^+ levels. • Very limited data base on ambient concentrations.
Ultrafine Particles ($D \leq 0.2\,\mu m$)	• Much greater potency per unit mass in animal inhalation studies (H^+ and TiO_2 aerosols) than for same materials in larger diameter fine particle aerosols. • Concept of "irritation signalling" in terms of number of particles per unit airway surface.	• Absence of relevant data on responses in humans. • Absence of relevant data base on ambient concentrations.

particles in the ultrafine mode (diameters below $50\,\mu m$), supported by animal work showing the ability of ultrafine particles of H_2SO_4 to cause death and other serious consequences at concentrations below $0.030\,\mu mg/m^3$. Alternatively, it may be that the combination of H^+ and ultrafines, i.e. acid-coated ultrafine particles, that might be important. Sulphuric acid coated on ultrafine zinc oxide particles produced similar responses, as did pure sulphuric acid, for a given

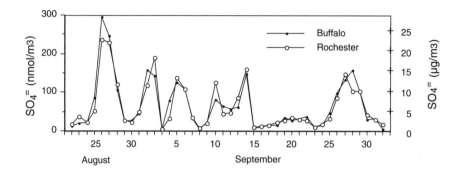

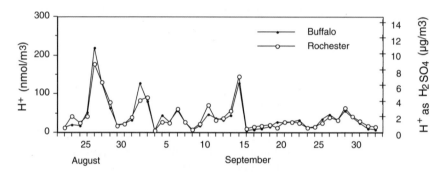

Fig. 6. Intercomparison of Rochester, NY and Buffalo, NY sulphate and daily acid aerosol concentrations (August 22 – October 2, 1990).

number of equivalent sized particles (Fig. 7); yet, the coated particles had only one-tenth of the acid content per unit volume of air. Thus, the response may be related to the number of acidic particles that deposit on the lung surfaces rather than the amount (mass) of acid deposited. In other words, the total concentration of H^+ may be a better surrogate of the active agent than $SO_4^=$ or $PM_{2.5}$, but it is still a crude index for the number concentration of irritant particles.

Finally, in the real world it is likely that the co-presence of acidity increases the solubility of toxic metals also present in ambient particles, thereby making these metals even more biologically-available to produce adverse oxidative stress responses. This may be an important pathway by which acidified particles, such as those resulting from fossil fuel burning power plant emissions of sulphur oxides, can have

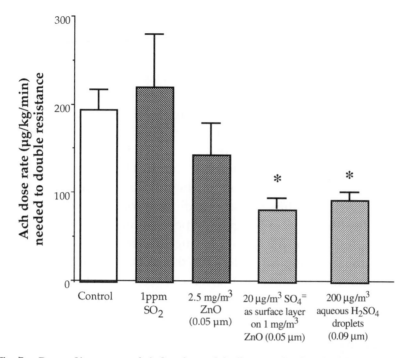

Fig. 7. Dose of intravenously infused acetylcholine required to double airway resistance in guinea pigs from baseline levels 2 hours after a 1 hour inhalation exposure. Values are mean ± S.E. The asterisks indicate reductions significant at $p < 0.05$. For the aerosols, the median particle diameters are indicated in parentheses.

heightened toxicity, and perhaps provide the most plausible physiological mechanism for explaining those epidemiological associations that have been found between acidic particle exposures and adverse human health effects.

8. Conclusion

Epidemiological evidence clearly suggests that acidic aerosols present during extreme pollution episodes are likely to have adverse health effects. Such evidence for effects at lower ambient levels is clouded by potential confounders, such as the presence of sulphur dioxide and other gaseous pollutants. While some epidemiological studies of sulphates and acidic aerosols suggest a potential role for acidic aerosols in PM-health effects associations, toxicological studies and controlled clinical studies with pure acidic particles have not been able to demonstrate adverse health outcomes at concentrations consistent with ambient levels, or even at much higher levels. However, such toxicological studies of pure acidic aerosols possibly do not replicate the way acidic aerosols are found in the atmosphere (e.g. as coatings on ambient particles containing other constituents, such as metals, with which they may interact). In addition, most toxicological studies used particles in the fine mode, and it is possible that effects noted in epidemiological studies, if due to H^+, were due to even smaller particles, perhaps those in the ultrafine mode. Thus, while epidemiological studies appear to indicate a role for acid aerosols in adverse health effects in the general population, and there is a plausible rationale for acidic species having adverse effects on biological systems, the toxicological evidence to date is inadequate in providing an indication of the specific mechanism for, or exact magnitude of any such effects on human health.

References

Amdur M.O. and Chen L.C. (1989) Furnace-generated acid aerosols: Speciation and pulmonary effects. *Environ Health Perspect* **79**: 147–150.

Amdur M.O., Sarofim A.F., Neville M., Quann R.J., McCarthy J.F., Elliott J.F., Lam H.F., Rogers A.E. and Conner M.W. (1986) Coal combustion aerosols and SO_2: An interdisciplinary analysis. *Environ Sci Technol* **20**: 138–145.

Aranyi C., Vana S.C., Thomas P.T., Bradof J.N., Fenters J.D., Graham J.A. and Miller F.J. (1983) Effects of subchronic exposure to a mixture of O_3, SO_2, and $(NH_4)2SO_4$ on host defenses of mice. *J Toxicol Environ Health* **12**(1): 55–71.

Avol E.L., Linn W.S., Wightman L.H., Whynot J.D., Anderson K.R. and Hackney J.D. (1988) Short-term respiratory effects of sulphuric acid in fog: A laboratory study of healthy and asthmatic volunteers. *J Air Pollut Control Assoc* **38**: 258–263.

Avol E.L. *et al.* (1988) Respiratory dose-response study of normal and asthmatic volunteers exposed to sulfuric acid aerosol in the sub-micrometer size range. *Toxicol Ind Health* **4**: 173–178.

Balmes J.R., Fine J.M., Christian D., Gordon T. and Sheppard D. (1988) Acidity potentiates bronchoconstriction induced by hypoosmolar aerosols. *Am Rev Respir Dis* **138**: 35–39.

Brauer M., Dumyahn T.S., Spengler J.D., Gutschmidt K., Heinrich J. and Wichmann H.E. (1995) Measurement of acidic aerosol species in Eastern Europe: Implications for air pollution epidemiology. *Environ Health Perspect* **103**: 482–488.

Brownstein D.G. (1980) Reflex-mediated desquamation of bronchiolar epithelium in guinea pigs exposed acutely to sulphuric acid aerosol. *Am J Pathol* **98**: 577–590.

Cavender F.L., Steinhagen W.H., Ulrich C.E., Busey W.M., Cockrell B.Y., Haseman J.K., Hogan M.D. and Drew R.T. (1977) Effects in rats and guinea pigs of short-term exposure to sulphuric acid mist, ozone, and their combination. *J Toxicol Environ Health* **3**: 521–533.

Charles J.M. and Menzel D.B. (1975) Ammonium and sulphate ion release of histamine from lung fragments. *Arch Environ Health* **30**: 314–316.

Chen L.C., Lam H.F., Kim E.J., Guty J. and Amdur M.O. (1990) Pulmonary effects of ultrafine coal fly ash inhaled by guinea pigs. *J Toxicol Environ Health* **29**: 169–184.

Chen L.C., Miller P.D. and Amdur M.O. (1989) Effects of sulphur oxides on eicosanoids. *J Toxicol Environ Health* **28**: 99–109.

Chen L.C., Miller P.D., Amdur M.O. and Gordon T. (1992) Airway hyperresponsiveness in guinea pigs exposed to acid-coated ultrafine particles. *J Toxicol Environ Health* **35**(3): 165–174.

Chen L.C., Miller P.D., Lam H.F., Guty J. and Amdur M.O. (1991) Sulphuric acid-layered ultrafine particles potentiate ozone-induced airway injury. *J Toxicol Environ Health* **34**: 337–352.

Chen L.C., Wu C.Y. and Qu Q.S. (1995) Number concentration and mass concentration as determinants of biological response to inhaled irritant particles. *Inhal Toxicol* **7**: 577–588.

Coggon D., Pannett B. and Wield G. (1996) Upper aerodigestive cancer in battery manufacturers and steel workers exposed to mineral acid mists. *Occ Environ Med* **53**: 445–449.

Commins B.T. and Waller R.E. (1967) Observations from a Ten-Year-Study of pollution at a site in the City of London. *Atmos Environ* **1**: 49–68.

Cookfair D., Wende K., Michalek A., *et al.* (1985) A case-control study of laryngeal cancer among workers exposed to sulphuric acid. *Am J Epidemiol* **122**: S21.

Damokosh A.I., Spengler J.D., Dockery D.W., Ware J.H. and Speizer F.E. (1993) Effects of acidic particles on respiratory symptoms in 7 U.S. Communities. *Am Rev Respir Dis* **147**: A632.

Dockery D.W., *et al.* (1996) Health effects of acid aerosols on North American children: Respiratory symptoms. *Environ Health Perspect* **104**: 500–505.

Dockery D.W., Schwartz J. and Spengler J.D. (1992) Air pollution and daily mortality: Associations with particulates and acid aerosols. *Environ Res* **59**: 362–373.

Dockery D.W., Pope C.A., Xu X., Spengler J.D., Ware J.H., Fay M.E., Ferris B.G. and Speizer F.E. (1993) An association between air pollution and mortality in six U.S. cities. *N Engl J Med* **329**: 1753–1759.

Dreher K.L., Jaskot R.J., Lehmann J.R., Richards J.H., McGee J.K., Ghio A.J. and Costa D.L. (1997) Soluble transition metals mediate residual oil fly ash induced acute lung injury. *J Toxicol Environ Health* **50**: 285–305.

el-Fawal H.A. and Schlesinger R.B. (1994) Nonspecific airway hyperresponsiveness induced by inhalation exposure to sulphuric acid aerosol: An *in vitro* assessment. *Toxicol Appl Pharmacol* **125**: 70–76.

Fine J.M., Gordon T., Thompson J.E. and Sheppard D. (1987) The Role of titratable acidity in acid aerosol-induced bronchoconstriction. *Am Rev Respir Dis* **135**: 826–830.

Firket M. (1931) Sur les causes des accidents survenus dans la vallée de la Meuse, lors des brouillards de décembre 1930 [The Causes of Accidents which Occurred in the Meuse Valley During the Fogs of December 1930]. *Bull Acad R Med Belg* **11**[ser. 5]: 683–741.

Frampton M.W., Voter K.Z., Morrow P.E., Roberts N.J. Jr., Culp D.J., Cox C. and Utell M.J. (1992) Effects of H_2SO_4 aerosol exposure in humans assessed by bronchoalveolar lavage. *Am Rev Respir Dis* **146**: 626–632.

Fujimaki H., Katayama N. and Wakamori K. (1992) Enhanced histamine release from lung mast cells of guinea pigs exposed to sulphuric acid aerosols. *Environ Res* **58**: 117–123.

Gearhart J.M. and Schlesinger R.B. (1986) Sulphuric-Acid induced airway hyperresponsiveness. *Fundam Appl Toxicol* **7**: 681–689.

Gearhart J.M. and Schlesinger R.B. (1988) Response of the tracheobronchial mucociliary clearance system to repeated irritant exposure: Effect of sulphuric acid mist on function and structure. *Exp Lung Res* **14**: 587–605.

Ghio A.J. and Devlin R.B. (2001) Inflammatory lung injury after bronchial instillation of air pollution particles. *Am J Respir Crit Care Med* **164**: 704–708.

Grose E.C., Gardner D.E. and Miller E.J. (1980) Response of ciliated epithelium to ozone and sulphuric acid, *Environ Res* **22**: 377–385.

Gwynn R.C., Burnett R.T. and Thurston G.D. (2000) A time-series analysis of acidic particulate matter and daily mortality and morbidity in the Buffalo, New York, region. *Environ Health Perspectives* **108**: 125–133.

Hattis D., Wasson J.M., Page G.S., Stern B. and Franklin C.A. (1987) Acid particles and the tracheobronchial region of the respiratory system: An "Irritation-Signaling" model for possible health effects. *J Air Pollut Control Assoc* **37**: 1060–1066.

Hemeon W.C.L. (1955) The estimation of health hazards from air pollution. *AMA Arch Ind Health* **11**: 397–402.

Holma B. (1985) Influence of buffer capacity and pH-dependent rheological properties of respiratory mucus on health effects due to acidic pollution. *Sci Total Environ* **41**: 101–123.

Holma B., Lindegran M. and Andersen J.M. (1977) pH effects on ciliomotility and morphology of respiratory mucosa. *Arch Environ Health* **32**: 216–226.

Ichinose T. and Sagai M. (1992) Combined exposure to nitrogen dioxide, ozone and sulphuric acid-aerosol and lung tumor formation in rats. *Toxicology* **74**: 173–184.

Ito K., Thurston G.D., Hayes C. and Lippmann M. (1993) Associations of London, England, daily mortality with particulate matter, sulphur dioxide, and acidic aerosol pollution. *Arch Environ Health* **48**: 213–220.

Kitagawa T. (1984) Cause analysis of the Yokkaichi asthma episode in Japan. *J Air Pollut Control Assoc* **34**: 743–746.

Kleinman M.T., McClure T.R., Mautz W.J. and Phalen R.F. (1985) The interaction of ozone and atmospheric acids on the formation of lung lesions in rats. In: Evaluation of the scientific basis for ozone/oxidants standards: Proceedings of an APCA International Specialty Conference, S.D. Lee, ed., November 1984; Houston, TX; Pittsburgh, PA: Air Pollution Control Association; pp. 357–365 (APCA Publication No. TR-4).

Knorst M.M., Kienast K., Riechelmann H., Muller-Quernheim J. and Ferlinz R. (1994) *In-vitro* evaluation of alterations in mucociliary clearance of guinea-pig tracheas induced by sulphur dioxide or nitrogen dioxide. *Pneumologie* **48**: 443–447.

Kobayashi T. and Shinozaki Y. (1993) Effects of exposure to sulphuric acid-aerosol on airway responsiveness in guinea pigs: Concentration and time dependency. *J Toxicol Environ Health* **39**: 261–272.

Koenig J.Q., Covert D.S., Larson T.V. and Pierson W.E. (1992) The effect of duration of exposure on sulphuric acid-induced pulmonary function changes in asthmatic adolescent subjects: A dose-response study. *Toxicol Ind Health* **8**: 285–286.

Koenig J.Q., Dumler K., Rebolledo V., Williams P.V. and Pierson W.E. (1993) Respiratory effects of inhaled sulphuric acid on senior asthmatics and non-asthmatics. *Arch Environ Health* **48**: 171–175.

Koenig J.Q., Pierson W.E. and Horike M. (1983) The effects of inhaled sulphuric acid on pulmonary function in adolescent asthmatics. *Am Rev Respir Dis* **128**: 221–225.

Larson T.V. (1993) Calculation of acid aerosol dose. in *Advances in Controlled Clinical Inhalation Studies*, ed. Mohr U., Springer-Verlag, Berlin, pp. 109–121.

Larson T.V., Covert D.S., Frank R. and Charlson R.J. (1977) Ammonia in the human airways: Neutralization of inspired acid sulphate aerosols. *Science* **197**: 161–163.

Larson T.V., Frank R., Covert D.S., Holub D. and Morgan M.S. (1982) Measurements of respiratory ammonia and the chemical neutralization of inhaled sulphuric acid aerosol in anesthetized dogs. *Am Rev Respir Dis* **125**: 502–506.

Last J.A., Hyde D.M. and Chang D.P. (1984) A mechanism of synergistic lung damage by ozone and a respirable aerosol. *Exp Lung Res* **7**: 223–235.

Laube B.L., Bowes S.M. 3rd, Links J.M., Thomas K.K. and Frank R. (1993) Acute exposure to acid fog: Effects on mucociliary clearance. *Am Rev Respir Dis* **147**: 1105–1111.

Lay J.C., Bennett W.D., Ghio A.J., Bromberg P.A., Costa D.L., Kim C.S., Koren H.S. and Devlin R.B. (1999) Cellular and biochemical response of the human lung after intrapulmonary instillation of ferric oxide particles. *Am J Respir Cell Mol Biol* **20**: 631–642.

Leikauf G., Yeates D.B., Wales K.A., Spektor D., Albert R.E. and Lippmann M. (1981) Effects of sulphuric acid aerosol on respiratory mechanics and mucociliary particle clearance in health nonsmoking adults. *Am Ind Hyg Assoc* **42**: 273–282.

Linn W.S., Avol E.L., Anderson K.R., Shamoo D.A., Peng R.C. and Hackney J.D. (1989) Effect of droplet size on respiratory responses to inhaled sulphuric acid in normal and asthmatic volunteers. *Am Rev Respir Dis* **140**: 161–166.

Linn W.S., Shamoo D.A., Anderson K.R., Peng R.C., Avol E.L. and Hackney J.D. (1994) Effects of prolonged, repeated exposures to ozone, sulphuric acid, and their combination in healthy and asthmatic volunteers. *Am J Respir Crit Care Med* **150**: 431–440.

Lioy P.J. and Waldman J.M. (1989) Acidic sulphate aerosols: Characterization and exposure. *Environ Health Perspect* **79**: 15–34.

Lippmann M. and Ito K. (1995) Separating the effects of temperature and season on daily mortality from those of air pollution in London: 1965–1972. in: *Proceedings of the Colloquium on Particulate Air Pollution and Human Mortality and Morbidity*, eds. Phalen R.F. and Bates D.V. (Irvine, CA, January 1994) *Inhal. Toxicol.* **7**: 85–97.

Lippmann M., Ito K., Nadas A. and Burnett R.T. (2000) Association of particulate matter components with daily mortality and morbidity in urban populations. *Res Rep Health Effect Inst* **95**: 5–72.

Mannix R.C., Mannix R.F., Phalen J.L., Kenoyer J.L. and Crocker T.T. (1982) Effect of sulphur dioxide-sulphate exposure on rat respiratory tract clearance. *Am Ind Hyg Assoc J* **43**: 679–685.

Martonen T.B. and Zhang Z. (1993) 'Deposition of sulphate aerosols in the developing human lung,' *Inhal Toxicol* **5** 165–187.

McGovern T.J. (1993) Effect of repeated *in vivo* ozone and/or sulphuric acid exposures on ß-adrenergic modulation of macrophage function. *Toxicologist* **13**: 49–52.

Morrow P.E. (1986) Factors determining hygroscopic aerosol deposition in airways,' *Physiol Rev* **66**: 330–376.

Nathanson I. and Nadel J.A. (1984) Movement of electrolytes and fluid across airways. *Lung* **162**: 125–137.

Neas L.M., Dockery D.W., Koutrakis P., Tollerud D.J. and Speizer F.E. (1995) The association of ambient air pollution with twice daily peak expiratory flow rate measurements in children. *Am J Epidemiol* **141**: 111–122.

Osebold J.W., Gershwin L.J. and Zee Y.C. (1980) Studies on the enhancement of allergic lung sensitization by inhalation of ozone and sulphuric acid aerosol. *J Environ Pathol Toxicol* **3**: 221–234.

Ostro B.D., Lipsett M.J., Wiener M.B. and Selner J.C. (1991) Asthmatic responses to airborne acid aerosols. *Am J Public Health* **81**: 694–702.

Peters A., Goldstein I.F., Beyer U., Franke K., Heinrich J., Dockery D.W., Spengler J.D. and Wichmann H.E. (1996) Acute health effects of exposure to high levels of air pollution in Eastern Europe. *Am J Epidemiol* **144**: 570–581.

Peto R., Speizer F.E., Cochrane A.L., Moore F., Fletcher C.M., Tinker C.M., Higgins I.T., Gray R.G., Richards S.M., Gilliland J. and Norman-Smith B. (1983) The relevance in adults of air-flow obstruction, but not of mucus hypersecretion, to mortality from chronic lung disease: Results from 20 years of prospective observation. *Am Rev Respir Dis* **128**: 491–500.

Phalen R.F., Kenoyer J.L., Crocker J.T. and McClure T.R. (1980) Effects of sulphate aerosols in combination with ozone on elimination of tracer particles by rats. *J Toxicol Environ Health* **6**: 797–810.

Pope C.A. III. (2000) Epidemiology of fine particulate air pollution and human health: Biologic mechanisms and who's at risk? *Environ Health Perspect* **108**(Suppl 4): 713–723.

Prasad S.B., Rao V.S., Mannix R.C. and Phalen R.F. (1988) Effects of pollutant atmospheres on surface receptors of pulmonary macrophages. *J Toxicol Environ Health* **24**(3): 385–402.

Prasad S.B., Rao V.S., McClure T.R., Mannix R.C. and Phalen R.F. (1990) Toxic effects of short-term exposures to acids and diesel exhaust. *J Aerosol Med* **3**: 147–163.

Qu Q.S., Chen L.C., Gordon T., Amdur M. and Fine J.M. (1993) Alteration of pulmonary macrophage intracellular pH regulation by sulphuric acid aerosol exposures. *Toxicol Appl Pharmacol* **121**: 138–143.

Raizenne M., Neas L.M., Damokosh A.I., Dockery D.W., Spengler J.D., Koutrakis P., Ware J.H. and Speizer F.E. (1996) Health effects of acid aerosols on North American children: Pulmonary function. *Environ Health Perspect* **104**: 506–514.

Riedel F., Kramer M., Scheibenbogen C. and Rieger C.H. (1988) Effects of SO_2 exposure on allergic sensitization in the guinea pig. *J Allergy Clin Immunol* **8**: 527–534.

Schiff L.J., Byrne M.M., Fenters J.D., Graham J.A. and Gardner D.E. (1979) Cytotoxic effects of sulphuric acid mist, carbon particulates and their mixtures on hamster tracheal epithelium. *Environ Res* **19**: 339–354.

Schlesinger R.B. (1984) Comparative irritant potency of inhaled sulphate aerosols — Effects on bronchial mucociliary clearance. *Environ Res* **34**: 268–279.

Schlesinger R.B. (1989) Factors affecting the response of lung clearance systems to acid aerosols: Role of exposure concentration, exposure time, and relative acidity. *Environ Health Perspect* **79**: 121–126.

Schlesinger R.B. (1990) The interaction of inhaled toxicants with respiratory tract clearance mechanisms. *Crit Rev Toxicol* **20**: 257–286.

Schlesinger R.B. (1995) The interaction of gaseous and particulate pollutants in the respiratory tract: Mechanisms and modulators. *Toxicology* **105**: 315–325.

Schlesinger R.B. and Chen L.C. (1994) Comparative biological potency of acidic sulphate aerosols: Implications for the interpretation of laboratory and field studies. *Environ Res* **65**: 69–85.

Schlesinger R.B., Gorczynski J.E., Dennison J., Richards L., Kinney P.L. and Bosland M.C. (1992) Long-term intermittent exposure to sulphuric acid aerosol, ozone, and their combination: Alterations in tracheobronchial mucociliary clearance and epithelial secretory cells. *Exp Lung Res* **18**: 505–534.

Schlesinger R.B., Gunnison A.F. and Zelikoff J.T. (1990) Modulation of pulmonary eicosanoid metabolism following exposure to sulphuric acid. *Fundam Appl Toxicol* **15**: 151–162.

Schlesinger R.B., Zelikoff J.T., Chen L.C. and Kinney P.L. (1992) Assessment of toxicologic interactions resulting from acute inhalation exposure to sulphuric acid and ozone mixtures. *Toxicol Appl Pharmacol* **115**: 183–190.

Schrenk H.H., Heineman H. and Clayton G.D. (1949) Air pollution in donora, PA. Epidemiology of the unusual smog episode of october 1948: Preliminary report. Washington, DC: Public health service, Public health service bulletin no. 306.

Schwartz J., Dockery D.W., Neas L.M., Wypij D., Ware J.H., Spengler J.D., Koutrakis P., Speizer F.E. and Ferris B.G. Jr. (1994) Acute effects of summer air pollution on respiratory symptom reporting in children. *Am J Respir Crit Care Med* **150**: 1234–1242.

Schwartz J., Wypij D., Dockery D., Ware J., Zeger S., Spengler J. and Ferris B. Jr. (1991) Daily diaries of respiratory symptoms and air pollution: Methodological issues and results. *Environ Health Perspect* **90**: 181–187.

Schwartz L.W., Moore P.F., Chang D.P., Tarkington B.K., Dungworth D.L. and Tyler W.S. (1977) Short-term effects of sulphuric acid aerosols on the respiratory tract. A morphological study in guinea pigs, mice, rats and monkeys. in: *Biochemical Effects of Environmental Pollutants*, ed. Lee S.D. (Ann Arbor Science, Ann Arbor), 257–271.

Silbaugh S.A., Mauderly J.L. and Macken C.A. (1981) Effects of sulphuric acid and nitrogen dioxide on airway responsiveness of the guinea pig. *J Toxicol Environ Health* **8**: 31–45.

Speizer F.E. (1989) Studies of acid aerosols in six cities and in a new multi-city investigation: Design issues. *Environ Health Perspectives* **79**: 61–67.

Spektor D.M., Leikauf G.D., Albert R.E. and Lippmann M. (1985) Effects of submicrometer sulphuric acid aerosols on mucociliary transport and respiratory mechanics in asymptomatic asthmatics. *Environ Res* **37**: 174–191.

Spektor D.M., Yen B.M. and Lippmann M. (1989) Effect of concentration and cumulative exposure of inhaled sulphuric acid on tracheobronchial particle clearance in healthy human. *Environ Health Perspect* **79**: 167–172.

Spengler J.D., *et al.* (1989) Exposures to acidic aerosols. in: Symposium on the health effects of acid aerosols, October 1987 (Research Triangle Park, NC). *Environ Health Perspect* **79**: 43–51.

Stengel P.W., Bendele A.M., Cockerham S.L. and Silbaugh S.A. (1993) Sulphuric acid induces airway hyperresponsiveness to substance P in the guinea pig. *Agents Actions* **39**: C128–131.

Thurston G.D., Ito K., Hayes C.G., Bates D.V. and Lippmann M. (1994) Respiratory hospital admissions and summertime haze air pollution in Toronto, Ontario: Consideration of the role of acid aerosols. *Environ Res* **65**: 271–290.

Thurston G.D., Ito K., Kinney P.L. and Lippmann M. (1992) A multi-year study of air pollution and respiratory hospital admissions in three New York state metropolitan areas: Results for 1988 and 1989 summers. *J Expos Anal Environ Epidemiol* **2**: 429–450.

Thurston G.D., Ito K., Lippmann M. and Hayes C. (1989) Reexamination of London, England, mortality in relation to exposure to acidic aerosols during 1963–1972 winters. in Symposium on the health effects of acid aerosols, October 1987 (Research Triangle Park, NC), *Environ Health Perspect* **79**: 73–82.

Tunnicliffe W.S., Mark D., Ayres J.G. and Harrison R.M. (2001) The effect of exposure to particulate sulphuric acid on the airway responses of mild atopic asthmatic subjects to inhaled grass pollen allergen. *Eur Resp J* 18: 640–647.

U.S. Environmental Protection Agency. An Acid Aerosols Issue Paper: Health Effects and Aerometrics. Office of Research and Development, Research Triangle Park, NC, Report No. EPA-600/8-88-005f; 1989.

United Kingdom Ministry of Health. Mortality and morbidity during the London fog of December 1952. (London, United Kingdom: Her majesty's stationery office, Reports on public health and medical subjects no. 95, 1954.)

Utell M.J., Margiglio J.A., Morrow P.E., Gibb F.R., Platner J. and Spears D.M. (1989) Effects of inhaled acid aerosols on respiratory function: The role of endogenous ammonia. *J Aerosol Med* 2: 141–147.

Utell M.J., Morrow P.E. and Hyde R.W. (1983) Latent development of airway hyper-reactivity in human subjects after sulphuric acid aerosol exposure. *J Aerosol Sci* 14: 202–205.

Veronesi B., Carter J.D., Devlin R.B., Simon S.A. and Oortgiesen M. (1999) Neuropeptides and capsaicin stimulate the release of inflammatory cytokines in a human bronchial epithelial cell line. *Neuropeptides* 33: 447–456.

Ward D., Roberts K., Jones N., Harrison R.M., Ayres J.G., Hussain S. and Walters S. (2002) Effects of daily variation in outdoor particulates and ambient acid species in normal and asthmatic children. *Thorax* 57: 489–502.

Warren D.L. and Last J.A. (1987) Synergistic interaction of ozone and respirable aerosols on rat lungs. III. ozone and sulphuric acid aerosol. *Toxicol Appl Pharmacol* 88: 203–216.

Wolff R.K. (1986) Effects of airborne pollutants on mucociliary clearance. *Environ Health Perspect* 66: 223–237.

Wolff R.K., Henderson R.F., Gray R.H., Carpenter R.L. and Hahn F.F. (1986) Effects of sulphuric acid mist inhalation on mucous clearance and on airway fluids of rats and guinea pigs. *J Toxicol Environ Health* 17: 129–142.

Zelikoff J.T. and Schlesinger R.B. (1992) Modulation of pulmonary immune defense mechanisms by sulphuric acid: Effects on macrophage-derived tumor necrosis factor and superoxide. *Toxicology* 76: 271–281.

Zelikoff J.T., Sisco M.P., Yang Z., Cohen M.D. and Schlesinger R.B. (1994) Immuno-toxicity of sulphuric acid aerosol: Effects on pulmonary macrophage effector and functional activities critical for maintaining host resistance against infectious diseases. *Toxicology* 92: 269–286.

CHAPTER 6

TESTING NEW PARTICLES

K. Donaldson, V. Stone, S. Faux and W. MacNee

1. Background to Particles and Lung Disease

This paper sets out possible approaches to the testing of novel particles whose toxicity is unknown. The strategy is based on a tiered system comprising:

(1) Characterisation of the particle for size and physico-chemistry
(2) Benchmarking against similar types of particle to anticipate the types of adverse pulmonary effects that might arise
(3) *In vitro* testing in relevant models
(4) Intratracheal and inhalation studies as necessary

There are a wide spectrum of different approaches to the testing of particles that range from long-term inhalation studies with the final endpoint of cancer, to short-term tests of the ability of the particle to modulate cellular functions. The value of each of these tests in predicting pathogenicity varies, but in general, there is a play-off between the extended time scale and high cost of a long-term pathogenicity experiments in animals which can be used in risk assessment, to the short time scale and relative cheapness of an *in vitro* experiment, which can, at best, be used in hazard assessment. If epidemiological or clinical evidence is available on the pathogenic outcome of exposure to the novel particle, then this would form the basis of a rational test strategy. However, as it is more likely for a novel particle, in the absence of such information, a strategy based on the knowledge of structure, chemistry and shape of the particle could allow benchmarking to similar particles of known pathogenicity in order to decide on the most appropriate endpoint.

1.1. *Which Particles Cause Lung Disease?*

Many particle types are known to cause lung disease. A selection of the best known are shown in Table 1, but this is incomplete and more thorough consideration of a wider range of particles is available in Morgan and Seaton (1995), and Churg and Green (1998). These shown in Table 1 are amongst the best understood as to their effects and mechanism of action and can act as benchmark particles in a preliminary consideration of likely pathogenic outcomes from exposure (see below).

1.2. *Which Diseases are Caused by Particles?*

Particle exposure is associated with a wide variety of pulmonary diseases, as shown in the Table 2.

For more detailed description of these and other particle-related lung diseases, see Morgan and Seaton (1995), Churg and Green (1998) and Parkes (1994). This spectrum of pathology poses an immediate problem for a testing strategy in that a strategy that is designed

Table 1.   Some particle types that are known to cause lung disease.

Particle
Asbestos
Quartz
Mixed dust e.g. coalmine dust
Nuisance dust e.g. carbon black
Metal dust e.g. nickel
Organic dust e.g. grain dust
Environmental particles ($PM_{2.5}$) e.g. diesel exhaust
Ultrafine particles

Table 2. Adverse health effects caused by exposure to different types of particles.

Disease	Exemplar Particles
Bronchitis	Coalmine dust, organic dust, PM_{10}
Small airways disease	Coalmine dust, quartz
Sensitisation/asthma	Metals, organic dusts
Emphysema	Coalmine dust, quartz
Fibrosis	Quartz, coalmine dust
Exacerbations of airways disease	$PM_{2.5}$
Stroke/ Heart attack	$PM_{2.5}$
Lung cancer	Quartz, metals, asbestos
Mesothelioma	Asbestos

to detect a carcinogenic endpoint, for example, would be entirely different from the one that would be chosen to the detect any potential in causing asthma. As such, there is a need for some knowledge of the likely pathology that would arise. This could be provided by:

(1) *A priori* knowledge from clinical observation or epidemiological study, indicating that a particular disease or manifestation of toxicity is associated with exposure to the particle.

(2) In the absence of such information, there could be benchmarking to particles such as those in Table 1. For example, if the particle type was a mineral and contained some quartz, then the endpoints of fibrosis and cancer could be selected; if the particle was organic or contained heavy metals, then sensitisation should be considered; and fibrous particles would be suspected of causing mesothelioma, etc.

1.3. *How Do Particles Cause Disease?*

The importance of inflammation

The ability to cause inflammation appears to be a central effector mechanism in the pathogenicity of particles (Fig. 1) and so tests aimed at determining the ability of particles to cause inflammation or

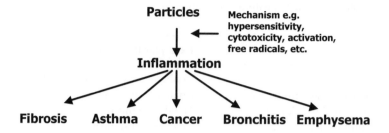

Fig. 1.   The central role of inflammation in the adverse health effects of particles.

to determine the pathways by which particles could elicit inflammation, either directly or indirectly, are an important part of any testing strategy.

While the detailed pathways that lead from the inflammation to the specific clinical endpoint are complex and often uncertain, the generic importance of inflammation can be recognised.

1.4. *Factors Affecting Particle Toxicity*

Particle size

Given the different diseases caused by particles, we can assume that there are different target cells and tissues (e.g. airways, alveolar cells, immune cells) that are affected by different particles. This is most easily understood from the point of view of differences in dose to these different target cells caused by differences in the distribution of dose throughout the respiratory tract because of variation in particle size. The fractional deposition of various sized particles for different pulmonary compartments is dictated by the aerodynamic diameter, D_{ae}, as shown in Fig. 2 and Table 3 (ISO, 1994). This is defined as the diameter of a particle of unit density with the same falling speed as the particle of interest.

Large particles > 20 μm D_{ae} only deposit in the upper respiratory tract, while particles from ~ 20 μm D_{ae} down to ~ 5 μm D_{ae}, deposit in the airways. Only particles smaller than ~ 5 μm D_{ae} deposit in the terminal airways and proximal alveoli, where the macrophages are responsible for defence. The net flow of air in this region is zero and so the very fine particles that can penetrate into this region

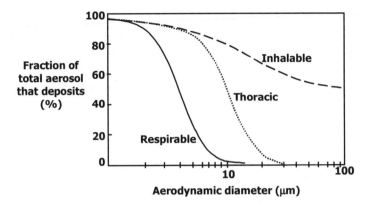

Fig. 2.   Deposition curves for particles of various aerodynamic diameter.

Table 3.   Anatomical site of deposition for the different deposition fractions.

Deposition Fraction	Definition	Site of Deposition
Inhalable	The fraction inhaled through the nose and mouth	Mouth, larynx, pharynx
Thoracic	Fraction penetrating beyond the larynx	The above plus airways
Respirable	Fraction penetrating beyond the ciliated airways	The above plus terminal bronchioles and alveolar ducts

can deposit by diffusion, a relatively efficient process (ISO, 1994). The macrophages, therefore, are responsible for phagocytosing and clearing a considerable burden of fine particles. There are, of course, differences in deposition between species because of the size and anatomy of the airspaces and this must be taken into account in determining the fractional deposition, and in designing the size distribution of the aerosol (Schlesinger *et al.*, 1998).

For instance, environmental airborne particles are currently measured in the UK, using an internationally approved measurement convention called PM_{10}. This sampler convention is a mass measure that replaced the "black smoke method", a reflectance method used until the end of the 80s. The PM_{10} sampler determines the mass of airborne particles in the size range that centres around 10 μm aerodynamic diameter. Thus, it samples a very low % of particles of 15 μm, 50% of particles 10 μm, ~ 80% of particles of 5 μm and > 90% of particles of 1 μm aerodynamic diameter. This is nearly equivalent to the "thoracic fraction" (ISO, 1994), defined as the mass fraction of airborne particles that penetrates beyond the larynx. As a mass measure, it does not take into account of the particle size, and so a given mass of very small particles, e.g. 0.1 μm diameter, contains far more particles by number than the same mass of 10 μm particles. As the principal target area for particle effects is beyond the ciliated airways, a finer fraction, close to the "respirable fraction" (ISO, 1994), is now being measured in the USA by the $PM_{2.5}$ sampling convention. This resulted from studies showing that this finer fraction is more closely associated with adverse health effects (Schwartz *et al.*, 1996; Peters *et al.*, 1997).

This foregoing discussion means that different-sized particles would be expected to elicit different types of pathogenic response, because they deposit in different regions, as shown in Table 4.

From the foregoing, it can be concluded that the characterisation of the size of a novel particle is important in deciding what is the most likely endpoint to examine, since size will bear directly on the site of deposition and its subsequent response. When the site of the adverse health effect is not the local lung environment, it is more difficult to know which site of deposition is most important, because there could be at least in theory translocation from any site of deposition; hence, the question marks over the site of deposition of particles

Table 4. The likely diseases resulting from different sizes of particles depositing in different compartments.

Deposition Site	Disease
Thoracic	Bronchitis, Asthma, Lung cancer, Exacerbations of airways disease
Respirable	Small airways disease, Emphysema, Fibrosis, Stroke/ Heart attack, Mesothelioma

that cause mesothelioma or are associated with strokes/heart attacks.

The example of ultrafine particles

Several toxicological studies have demonstrated the increased toxicity of ultrafine particles i.e. particles of < 100nm diameter, compared with fine particles of the same material (reviewed in Donaldson *et al.*, 1998). Particles such as carbon and TiO_2 which are non-toxic as respirable, but non-ultrafine particles have been shown to have toxicity when they are in the form of ultrafine particles (Donaldson *et al.*, 1998). The ultrafine particles component of air pollution particles ($PM_{10}/PM_{2.5}$) has been hypothesised to be the main mediator of the adverse health effect (Seaton *et al.*, 1995; Donaldson and MacNee, 1998). As particle size become smaller, for any given mass of particles, the particle number increases dramatically and the total particle surface area also increases. High numbers of ultrafine particles are therefore likely to present a substantial problem for the macrophage defences, as they attempt to phagocytose them and keep the epithelium free of particles. Ultrafine particles may also be taken up rapidly by epithelial cells, because of their small size and their surface characteristics.

The surface of particles or substances that are released from the surface, e.g. transition metals, are the chemical structures that interact with the biological system. For "non-toxic" materials such as carbon and titanium dioxide, the effective dose i.e. the dose that mediates toxicity, appears to be a function of surface area. This is demonstrated by the fact that, for a range of fine and ultrafine-sized preparations of these materials, the inflammatory response was best related to particle surface area (Oberdorster, 1996) and the threshold surface area for overload with non-toxic particles is 200--300 cm^2 (Tran *et al.*, 1998). Furthermore, Driscoll (1996a) examined a large series of data on overload tumours caused by non-toxic dusts, titanium dioxide, diesel soot, carbon black, photocopier toner, talc and coalmine dust. In this series, the surface area of particulate in the lung was the best correlate of tumorigenicity, and not particle mass.

The central role of particle surface provides the basis for a hypothesis of toxicity based on the presence of surface-associated free radicals or free radical-generating systems. Transition metal-generated oxidants derived from the particle surface are considered to play an important role in the cytotoxic and cell-stimulating effects of a range of particles such as asbestos (Simeonova and Luster, 1995), quartz (Castranova *et al.*, 1996), residual oil fly ash (Dreher *et al.*, 1997) and PM_{10} (Gilmour *et al.*, 1996). If ultrafine particles were to cause toxicity by e.g. a transition metal-mediated mechanism or via a reactive surface, their relatively large surface area could mean severe oxidative stress to cells that they were in contact with. Macrophages would be subjected to oxidative stress during their attempts to phagocytose particles and could be oxidatively damaged or stimulated to release pro-inflammatory cytokines via oxidative stress-responsive transcription factors (Rahman and MacNee, 1998).

The large numbers of ultrafine particles depositing per unit mass means that substantial numbers of particles would evade macrophage phagocytosis. The unphagocytosed particles would then undergo more prolonged interaction with epithelial cells that could lead to epithelial cell oxidative stress, secretion and epithelial permeability and/or injury, which could enhance the interstitialisation of the ultrafine particles (Donaldson *et al.*, 1998).

Particle shape

The example of fibres

Particles come in a number of different shapes e.g. compact, platy (i.e. flat, flaky and soft) and fibrous. The importance of particle shape is best understood for fibres and fibre length is known to be a major factor in pathogenicity (Stanton *et al.*, 1981). Long fibres of amosite asbestos were much more pathogenic than a sample of the same material milled, so the fibre length was drastically shortened, with much of the sample being so short that it was classified as non-fibrous (Davis *et al.*, 1986). For other particles, shape is less obvious as a parameter that mediates toxicity. Shape may not be the only factor that dictates fibre pathogenicity, since even among long, thin fibres, there are differences in pathogenicity, especially in mesothelioma production. Erionite (Maltoni *et al.*, 1982) and Silicon carbide fibres (Davis *et al.*, 1996), for example, were much more active in causing mesothelioma following inhalation exposure than would be expected from their dimensions. For this reason, it is likely that another factor, surface reactivity (see below), could be important in mediating some of their pathogenicity (Brown *et al.*, in press).

Particle surface reactivity

The example of quartz

One of the most toxic particles is quartz and it is known to have a highly reactive surface. The quartz surface can generate reactive species in several ways following interactions of the quartz particles with pulmonary cells or lung fluids. Silanol groups (Si–OH) and ionised silanol groups (Si–O–) on the surface interact with membranes (Castranova *et al.*, 1995). The regular Si/O tetrahedra are interrupted when the quartz is cracked to form respirable particles, producing both homolytic and heterolytic cleavage of the Si-O bonds that make up the basic crystalline structure of the quartz (Fubini *et al.*, 1995). Homolytic cleavage results in Si• and Si–O• radicals, while heterolytic cleavage produces charged Si+ and Si–O– groups and these are present on the fractures surface of the quartz particles. In lung lining fluid or in tissue fluid, the products of homolytic cleavage can give rise to OH• and H_2O_2 (Castranova *et al.*, 1995), while the charged products of heterolytic cleavage are involved in interactions with membranes (Fubini *et al.*, 1995). Contaminating metals such as iron and aluminium (Guthrie and Heaney, 1995) may lower the toxicity of quartz, but Fenton chemistry-derived hydroxyl radicals may also be generated (Castranova *et al.*, 1996), adding to the oxidative stress.

Particle-derived transition metals

The example of transition metals in PM_{10} and other pollution particles

The relatively high iron content of some pneumoconiotic dusts (Kennedy *et al.*, 1989) raises the possibility that iron may be important in mediating the harmful effects of a range of particles. Iron has the ability to generate free radicals via Fenton chemistry that is well characterised. The state of the iron is all important, in particular, the amount of Fe(ll) is central since this is the directly harmful species. Consequently, total iron is not necessarily informative as to the biologically active iron. The iron must redox-cycle to be able to cause major injury to macromolecules, and this is accomplished by a reductant in the region of the particle e.g. glutathione, ascorbate, NADH or even superoxide anion. This means that the presence of anti-oxidants in the inflammatory milieu is a double-edged sword (see above).

By the sequence of events shown in Fig. 3, the highly toxic hydroxyl radical can be formed. The hydroxyl radical may be involved in diffusion-limited reactions which leads to the formation of various carbon-centred radicals, peroxyl, alkoxyl and thiyl radicals, all of which have harmful consequences for cells. As different reductants could have different potencies in causing reduction of Fe(III), and because of the known role of the chelating agents, the microenvironment of the lung where the fibre is present could be most important in determining how much reactive iron is present on the

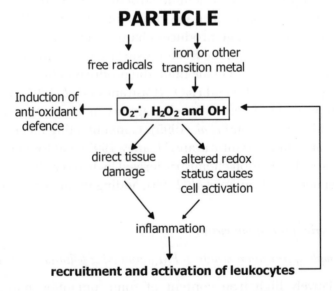

Fig. 3.   Generation of oxidative stress by particles.

fibre surface. In addition, the particle may accumulate biological iron which can also have free radical-generating activity (Lund *et al.*, 1994; Ghio *et al.*, 1994). In various models, the biological effects of several different types of ambient particle, including PM_{10} and ROFA, have been suggested to be driven by their transition metals content (Gilmour *et al.*, 1996; Dreher *et al.*, 1995; Kodavanti *et al.*, 1997; Carter *et al.*, 1997).

Particle biopersistence

Biopersistence is the capacity for particle to survive unchanged in the lungs. Biopersistence is limited by the potential of particles to dissolve or lose elements, break or be mechanically cleared from the lungs by macrophages. The potential for a particle to survive unchanged in the lungs would seem intuitively to be an important factor, since the dose of particle would not be expected to build up in the case of biopersistent particle. However, little is know about the biochemical conditions that pertain in the lungs and so the lung is largely a "black box" in this regard, although differences in pH and the impact of coating of the particles is to be anticipated.

The best case where this property is seen as being important is with fibres. Long fibres are not well cleared from the respiratory region of the lungs (Coin *et al.*, 1994), presumably because of the difficulties of the alveolar macrophage to successfully phagocytose and then move with them to the mucociliary escalator. Thus, the ability of long fibres to persist in the lungs without being either dissolved away or weakened so that they break into smaller fibres which can be easily cleared, is seen as an important factor contributing to pathogenicity (Hesterberg *et al.*, 1994).

In the case of particles, solubility is also an important factor that will influence the lung dose at any point during ongoing exposure, since the retained particles will be calculated as follows:

Retained mass or dose = (mass deposited)

$$- (\text{mass cleared} + \text{mass dissolved}).$$

If we assume two particles of equal diameter and density, one of which is soluble and one is not, then the particle that is soluble will not contribute to the dose as much as the non-soluble particle. The exception to this is the situation where a particle in the act of dissolving releases compounds and elements that have some intrinsic toxicity e.g. heavy metals. In this case, dissolution may be a factor that contributes to toxicity. The result of the combination of chemical dissolution, breakage of the particles and "mechanical" clearance by the macrophages is termed "biopersistence". Biopersistence may be dominated by mechanical clearance in the case of a non-soluble particle or there may be a variable contribution of chemical dissolution and breakage for particles of differing solubility and shape. Shape is a factor since a long thin fibre, which has undergone partial dissolution, may have weakness that, along with the forces acting along the length of the fibre in the lung milieu, may lead to breakage more readily than it would have been seen with a compact particle. From the foregoing, we would anticipate that non-durable fibres would be less pathogenic than durable ones (Warheit *et al.*, 1993).

2. Approaches to Testing

2.1. *Characterising the Particles*

An understanding of the nature of the particles with regard to shape, size, elemental composition, transition metal content, endotoxin contamination, etc is vital (see above). However, there are a huge number of parameters that could be assessed. Once again, the concept of benchmarking is a useful one and the source of the particle e.g. mineral–derived, man-made fibre, ash etc. can be used to decide which is the most likely parameter to be determined. Table 5 shows some particle characteristics that can be quantified, that might shed light on the likely pathogenicity of a particle sample.

Endotoxin is a potential confounder in all studies with particles and its presence should be rigorously monitored, since it may explain all the toxicity of a dust sample (e.g. Brown and Donaldson, 1996).

Samples to be used in testing

Care should be taken in the strategy for preparing the batch of material for testing. As particles can have their toxicity altered rather easily

Table 5. Important particle characteristics that can be measured in a sample of particles of unknown toxicity.

		Particle	Type	
	Mineral	**Combustion Particle**	**Ash**	**Fibre**
Dimensions	✓	✓	✓	✓
Surface area/ unit mass	✓	✓	✓	✓
Quartz/ cristobalite	✓		✓	
Heavy metals		✓	✓	
Transition metals	✓	✓	✓	✓
Bio-persistence	✓	✓	✓	✓
Free radical activity	✓	✓	✓	✓
PAH		✓		✓
Biopersistence	✓	✓	✓	✓
Endotoxin	✓	✓	✓	✓

by changing the way that the samples are prepared, or because the particles have different origins, the nature of the "stock" sample should be given careful consideration. The bulk material is best prepared in a single batch, well mixed and stored in a way that preserves the particles. Making new batches carries a risk that difference will arise in preparation or origin of the source material, that leads to difference in toxicity between the batches. Samples should be tested for endotoxin (see below).

2.2. *Assessment of Toxicity In Vitro*

The European Centre for the Validation of Alternative Methods recently published a report on "Non-animal tests for evaluating the toxicity of solid xenobiotics" and this contains recommendations for *in vitro* test with particles (Fubini *et al*, 1998). The majority of *in vitro* tests for detecting particle toxicity are aimed at detecting either direct or indirect pro-inflammatory effects. Acute and chronic inflammation is thought to be central to the aetiology of many lung disorders, such as asthma and chronic obstructive pulmonary disease (COPD). The specific characteristics of the inflammatory response may be different, but all are characterised by the recruitment of inflammatory cells into the lung. These activated cells, such as alveolar macrophages, produce cytokines and reactive oxygen species (ROS), and many other mediators involved in inflammation. Once triggered, the inflammatory response will persist in these conditions, leading to subsequent lung injury. The intracellular mechanism in the lung epithelium, and the macrophages leading to lung injury in response to environmental particulates, will involve the activation and upregulation of transcription factors such as activator protein-1 (AP-1) and nuclear factor-κB (NF-κB), leading to increased gene expression and the biosynthesis of proinflammatory mediators (Rahman and MaNee, 1998).

Using the tiered approach to the testing of a new particle, *in vitro* models provide a useful tool at two stages, namely the assessment of toxicity and the elucidation of their mechanism of action. A reduction in the use of experimental animals is a clear advantage of such studies, but *in vitro* systems also provide a "simplified" model in which the details of the mechanism of action may be readily probed.

The potential toxicity of particles is easily tested *in vitro* using either primary cells or cell lines in culture. There are a number of cell types which are of obvious interest when investigating the potential effects of particles, including type I and type II epithelial cells, Clara cells, alveolar macrophages and neutrophils. Primary cells are obviously an advantage in that they are not transformed, and hence will correspond more closely to the cells found *in vivo*. Despite this, cell lines such as the A549 human type II cell line and THP-1 monocytes, are widely used due to their ready availability and the fact that the pathways under study are similar in these permanent cell lines to freshly-derived cells of the same type. The acquisition of human primary cells remains difficult for many researchers, for this reason, rat primary cells are frequently used as an alternative. The use of cell lines has both benefits and drawbacks which are well known. The benefits include the ability to dissect out the sub-cellular pathways and responses, and to isolate the responses specific to the cell type in question. The drawbacks are that there is no influence of the other cell types and the circulation that ordinarily play an important role in the the responses of any single cell type.

Measuring cytotoxicity

In order to ascertain the potential for particles to induce patho-logical damage *in vivo*, comparative testing of different particles to induce cell death or decreased viability *in vitro* is required. A number of reliable and well documented techniques are available to assess viability, including the MTT assay (Mossman, 1983; measurement of succinate dehydrogenase enzyme activity and hence metabolic com-petence) and assessment of lactate dehydrogenase (LDH) enzyme leakage from the cells (Korzeniewski and Callewaert, 1983). The MTT assay and measurement of LDH leakage are appropriate for death via necrosis. A number of particle types have been proposed to induce programmed cell death or apoptosis (Iyer *et al.*, 1996; BeruBe *et al.*, 1996). The techniques available for the detection of apoptosis are numerous, from detection of DNA fragmentation to commercially available cell death ELISA kits and fluorescent dyes, such as propid-ium iodide and Hoechst 33342 that label the DNA.

Measurement of cell stimulation in vitro

Many particles are thought to induce effects on the lung by mecha-nisms other than toxicity. Some particles may in fact cause the stim-ulation of various cell types by e.g. increasing entry of calcium or stimulating kinase activity, leading to cell proliferation or an increase in the production of cytokines and other pro-inflammatory media-tors. Measurement of the production of ROS and cytokines, such as TNF-α and IL-1β, by target cells may form part of a testing strategy to discriminate between non-pathogenic and pathogenic particu-lates by the ability of various particulate preparations to differen-tially produce these mediators. There are a number of assays that can be used to assess cell stimulation *in vitro* and these are outlined below.

Cell proliferation measurement

Increased cell proliferation has been noted on exposure of various cell types to different particles. For example, treatment of primary rat type II epithelial cells with silica for 24 hours has been shown to induce cell proliferation, as assessed by the incorporation of tritiated thymidine into the DNA of dividing cells (e.g. Melloni *et al.*, 1996). This simple technique has the disadvantage of using radioactivity, although of a low level. A similar technique involves the incorporation of 5-bromo-2'-deoxyuridine (BrdU) into DNA, which is then assessed by immunostaining (e.g. Timblin *et al.*, 1995). This non-radioactive technique has the advantage that BrdU can be used for both observation by microscopy, as well as quantification through either spectroscopy or fluorimetery.

Techniques used to assess proliferation also reveal decreased proliferation. In addition, some assays which are used to assess cytotoxicity can be used to study proliferation, for example, the MTT assay mentioned above. An increase in the production of coloured formazan product from tetrazolium salts such as MTT can be used as an indicator of cell number (Berridge *et al.*, 1996).

Cytokine measurement

One of the most obvious ways to assess the potential inflammogenic activity of a particle is by measuring the output of cytokines. Secreted cytokines are frequently assayed in the culture media through the use of ELISA and in the case of TNFα, also by the use of cell assays (e.g. Brown and Donaldson, 1996). In addition, the quantification of specific mRNA sequences through either Northern Blotting or RT-PCR allows further investigation of gene regulation on exposure to particles. The same techniques are also applicable to other pro-inflammatory mediators.

Oxidative stress measurement

There is abundant data to suggest that many particle types induce their effects on the lungs in part through ROS and oxidative stress (reviewed in Donaldson, 1998). The free radicals produced at the surface of a variety of particle types, along with the reactive oxygen species released by leukocytes during phagocytosis and inflammation, induce an oxidative stress within the lung, leading to a range of events from oxidative damage to bio-molecules to activation of oxidative stress-responsive transcription factors that lead to transcription of pro-inflammatory genes (Rahman and MacNee, 1998). The measurement of intracellular glutathione in its reduced (GSH) and oxidised (GSSG) forms remains a sensitive means by which the induction of oxidative stress can be assessed. GSH is one of the major intracellular antioxidants (reviewed in Droge *et al.*, 1994). In acting as an antioxidant, two molecules of GSH are oxidised to form GSSG, which is then reduced back to GSH by the enzyme glutathione reductase using NADPH as a source of reductant. When the cell is exposed to high levels of oxidants, NADPH within the cell is decreased allowing depletion of GSH and an increase in GSSG. The depletion of GSH is often used as a marker of oxidative stress in response to particles (e.g. Stone *et al.*, 1998). For example, ultrafine CB (14 nm diameter; $0.78 \, \mu g/mm^2$) has been shown to induce a depletion of intracellular GSH in the human type II epithelial cell line A549 within 6 hours of exposure (Stone *et al.*, 1998). Non-pathogenic carbon black of larger diameter (260 nm) did not induce any significant depletion of cellular GSH over 8 hours of exposure. An increase in GSSG is often more difficult to establish (Stone *et al.*, 1998). GSSG is toxic to the cell due to its ability to form disulphide bonds with thiol groups, hence it is rapidly excreted from the cell (Chabot *et al.*, 1998). For this reason, measurement of an increase in intracellular GSSG as a marker for oxidative stress may be difficult.

When GSH levels are depleted within the cell, the enzymes responsible for GSH synthesis are often up-regulated, causing the GSH levels to increase above their original control values (Liu *et al.*, 1996). Enzyme assays exist to measure the activity of enzymes such as γ-glutamyl transpeptidase (γ-GT), the enzyme responsible for the uptake of the components of GSH across the plasma membrane and γ-glutamylcysteine synthetase (γ-GCS), the rate limiting enzyme in the synthesis of GSH. In addition, transfection of cell lines with a plasmid containing the promoter regions of the genes encoding for these enzymes provide a useful tool to study the up-regulation of these genes by oxidants (Rahman *et al.*, 1996).

Altered cell signalling on exposure to particles

Alterations in intracellular calcium

Alterations in intracellular calcium homeostasis have been implicated in oxidative stress. In the resting non-stimulated cell, a Ca^{2+}ATPase pump in the plasma membrane actively extrudes Ca^{2+} from the cell, while a different Ca^{2+}ATPase pump in the endoplasmic reticulum (ER) actively sequesters Ca^{2+} into this intracellular store. The ER Ca^{2+} store is released on activation of the cell by stimulants, which resulted in the production of inositol 1,4,5-trisphosphate (IP_3) (Chow *et al.*, 1995). This sharp increase in cytosolic calcium concentration stimulates the opening of Ca^{2+} channels in the plasma membrane (calcium release activated calcium channels; CRAC channels), allowing Ca^{2+} to enter the cell and down its concentration gradient (calcium release activated calcium current, I_{CRAC}), resulting in a sustained increase in cytosolic Ca^{2+} concentration (Parekh and Penner, 1997). A number of the transport proteins involved in the maintenance of Ca^{2+} homeostasis are sensitive to oxidative stress. For example, the Ca^{2+}-ATPase of the ER contains a cysteine residue which is susceptible to oxidation, as do the IP_3 receptor calcium channels in the ER (Berridge, 1993).

Cytosolic Ca^{2+} can be measured using fluorescent dyes such as fura-2 (Grynkiewicz *et al.*, 1985) which alter their fluorescent properties on binding to Ca^{2+}. Fura-2 has the advantage of being a ratio dye, which permits alterations in background fluorescence, for example, due to the introduction of particles, while measuring calcium.

UfCB ($66 \mu g/ml$) has been shown to increase the resting cytosolic calcium concentration of a human monocytic cell line MonoMac 6 (MM6) (Stone *et al.*, submitted for publication). This effect was not observed with the same dose of larger, respirable CB particles nor with pathogenic α-quartz (DQ12). Higher doses of silica have been reported elsewhere to induce an increase in the cytosolic Ca^{2+} concentration of macrophages (Lim *et al.*, 1997; Chen *et al.*, 1991).

A useful tool to investigate the potential effects of particles on Ca^{2+} signalling is thapsigargin (Thastrup *et al.*, 1990). Thapsigargin works by inhibiting the ER Ca^{2+}ATPase, resulting in the leak of the ER store contents into the cytosol. Treatment with thapsigargin results in a sharp increase in cytosolic Ca^{2+} (comparable to the effect of IP_3), followed by a stimulation of the I_{CRAC}. Treatment of a macrophage cell line (MonoMac 6) with ufCB for 30 minutes induced a 2.6-fold increase in the I_{CRAC} observed on treatment with thapsigargin, through increased opening of the plasma membrane Ca^{2+} channels (Stone *et al.*, submitted for publication). The amplification of second messenger signals on interaction with stimuli such as LPS (Carter *et al.*, 1998) or $TNF\alpha$ (Peces and Urra, 1995) could lead to an exaggerated activation of specific transcription factors, and hence genes encoding for pro-inflammatory factors.

This amplification and effects described above have recently been observed in rat pleural mesothelial cells exposed to mineral particles. In these studies, co-treatment of cells with NIEHS crocidolite asbestos and thapsigargin synergistically increased message levels of the proto-oncogene c-fos above that are seen with either agent alone (Faux *et al.*, submitted for publication). Using calcium chelators, the effect on gene expression was concluded to be due to an influx of extracellular calcium, due in turn to the exposure to the asbestos. In these experiments, thapsigargin caused calcium to be released from the ER stores and crocidolite caused calcium to enter the cell from the extracellular medium through increased opening of plasma membrane calcium channels. The results of such studies imply that particles may not provide a direct stimulus for the cells, but "prime" them so that they respond to subsequent physiological stimuli in an exaggerated manner. This has obvious implications for protocols to investigate the mechanism of action of particles. Sequential- and co-treatments with particles and cytokines would provide answers to some of these questions.

In contrast, exposure of human white blood cells to UICC crocidolite asbestos induced a depletion of the thapsigargin-releasable stores (Faux *et al.*, 1994). Such changes have been suggested elsewhere to be related to the induction of apoptosis (McConkey and Orrenius, 1997).

Mitogen-activated protein kinase (MAPK)

The MAPK cascade includes the extracellular signal-related kinase (ERK1, ERK2) activated in response to growth factors or phorbol esters via a Ras-dependent mechanism, c-Jun amino terminal kinase/stress activated protein kinase (JNK1, JNK2) activated by TNF-α in a Ras-independent manner and p38 (Seger and Krebb, 1995). Activation of the MAPK cascade involving phosphorylation and dephosphorylation of a number of proteins, leads to the transactivation of c-fos and c-jun and a number of interrelated transcription factors (Karin, 1995; Seger and Krebbs, 1995). Activation of JNK causes phosphorylation of Jun (Baker *et al.*, 1992) and ERKs phophorylate and potentiate the transactivation of c-fos (Janknecht *et al.*, 1995). Moreover, in a number of cellular systems, the balance between the activation of several arms of this pathway appears to govern, whether apoptosis or cell proliferation occurs (Xia *et al.*, 1995).

Limited studies have been carried out investigating the influence of particulates on the MAPK pathway. One recent study has shown that particulate matter causes activation of the JNK cell signalling cascade, after uptake or interaction with rat lung epithelial (RLE) cells. Timblin *et al.* (1998) show in these studies that exposure of RLE cells to particulate matter leads to the phosphorylation of c-Jun, and the transcriptional activation of AP-1 regulated genes lead to cell proliferation.

Transcription factor activation

ROS and inflammatory cytokines both cause activation of the transcription factors NF-κB and AP-1 (Meyer *et al.*, 1993). In addition, ROS have been suggested to act as second messenger molecules within the cell (Sen and Packer, 1996). The transcription factors NF-κB and AP-1 have been shown to be regulated by the intracellular redox status. Both transcription factors possess a cysteine thiol group, the oxidation of which leads to the activation of NF-κB and its translocation to the nucleus (Sen and Packer, 1996).

NF-κB is a transcription factor important in the regulation of a number of genes intrinsic to inflammation, proliferation and lung defences (Thanos and Maniatis, 1995), including cytokines, nitric oxide synthase, adhesion molecules and protooncogenes, such as c-myc. Protein subunits that bind to nuclear NF-κB elements are members of the Rel family of genes and occur in the cytoplasm of the cell bound to the inhibitory protein (IκB). The process of NF-κB activation involves the cytoplasmic phosphorylation, ubiquitination and subsequent proteolytic degradation of the IκB inhibitory subunits from NF-κB (Palombella *et al.*, 1994; Israel, 1995). Release of NF-κB from IκB allows uncovering of the nuclear localisation site on the NF-κB subunits so that it can migrate to the nucleus. Once in the nucleus, the activated transcription factor complex which include p65 protein subunits (Schmitz and Baeuerle, 1991) then bind to promoter regions of genes that have consensus NF-κB DNA binding sequences, such as c-myc (LaRosa *et al.*, 1994) and nitric oxide synthase (Xie *et al.*, 1994).

AP-1 is a family of accessory transcription factors that interact with other regulatory sequences known as TPA-response element (TRE) or AP-1 sites (Angel and Karin, 1991). AP-1 transcription factors include homo- (Jun/Jun) and heterodimer (Fos/Jun) complexes encoded by various members of the c-fos and c-jun families of protooncogenes. The functional ramifications of c-fos and c-jun transactivation may be cell type specific, but Fos and Jun proteins may regulate the expression of other genes required for the progression through the cell cycle, apoptosis or cell transformation (Angel and Karin, 1991).

It has been demonstrated in a number of cell types that asbestos fibres increase DNA binding activities of AP-1 (Heintz *et al.*, 1993; Howden and Faux, 1997) and NF-κB (Gilmour *et al.*,1997; Howden and Faux, 1997) and transactivation of AP-1 (Timblin *et al.*, 1995) and NF-κB (Janssen *et al.*, 1995) dependent gene expression. More recently, Quay *et al.* (1998) have demonstrated that residual oil fly ash (ROFA) can also increase the DNA binding of NF-κB in bronchial epithelial cells. Simeonova and Luster (1996), using A549 cells transfected with a construct containing the IL-8 gene promoter region, were able to show that crocidolite asbestos induced a binding of nuclear proteins to the NF-κB binding site of the IL-8 promoter. In addition, recent studies using ambient particulate matter showed transcriptional activation of AP-1 dependent genes in RLE cells (Timblin et al., 1998).

NF-κB binds to the promoter for the gene encoding IκB, leading to an increase in the transcription and translation of this inhibitory subunit. The resultant protein is able to enter the nucleus and bind to NF-κB, resulting in its dissociation from DNA and relocation into the cytoplasm. IκB protein levels can be assessed by western blotting. Recent data (Schins et al., 1998) suggests that different particle types vary in their affects on the level of IκB expressed in A549 cells. The differences between ultrafine and larger respirable particles remain yet to be fully elucidated. Activation of transcription factors can be investigated via a number of methods including the gel mobility assays of transcription factor DNA binding, immunohistochemical analysis of cellular localisation, gene transactivation assay using reporter constructs and western blotting of protein levels.

In vitro tests for genotoxicity

The recognition of carcinogenesis as the complex culmination of DNA damage, repair, mutations that are both chromosomal and at the gene level, DNA methylation, signal transduction, translation, etc means that there is a large battery of tests that can be used to detect the ability of particles to cause cancer. Indeed, there is some overlap with pro-inflammatory tests described above, since inflammation may play a key role in carcinogenesis of some particles such as quartz (e.g. Donaldson and Borm, 1998). The types of test available include assays of mammalian cell transformation, DNA breaks, oxidative adducts of DNA, micronucleus assay and inhibition of DNA repair. These assays are reviewed extensively in Fubini et al. (1998) with regard to their use for detecting particle effects. It is important to note that the carcinogenic effects detected for a number of particles in animal models, e.g. quartz, and some non-toxic particles at overload, are a consequence of inflammation and so they would not be detected by "classical" assays of genotoxicity.

2.3. *Animal Studies*

Rats are the "gold standard" in toxicology studies and rats are used extensively to study particle effects. The issue of overload must however be kept in mind (see below) when considering the exposure, and instillation studies should also be interpreted with care. There is a movement towards replacement of animals with human test systems and that remains an important goal.

Intratracheal instillation

In instillation, a mass of the particle sample is instilled into the lungs of anaesthetised rats in a small volume of saline. Although instillation has a number of problems because of the high dose and high dose rate delivered in the bolus, this technique has value in comparing between particle samples. The technique is more problematic for fibres, which tend to clump and bridge small airways leading to granulomas in the airspaces. However, a comparison between instillation and inhalation for particles has demonstrated that the same types of qualitative response were seen (Henderson *et al.*, 1995). The technique can be used for histopathology studies, but it is more often used in combination with BAL to study the short to medium-term inflammatory response to a suspect particle, in relation to a known pathogenic particle such as quartz and a non-pathogenic particle such as pigment grade TiO_2 (e.g. Zhang *et al.*, 1998). There is a distinct problem of "local overload" of lung defences when non-toxic particles are used in this assay, thus it is best used in comparison studies for toxic particles with the inclusion of relevant controls.

Inhalation studies

Inhalation studies are commonly carried out in conventional toxicology protocols to determine the likely toxicity of particles. Rats are maintained in chambers that deliver either whole body or nose-only exposure to clouds of particles conventionally, for up to 7 hours per day, 5 days per week (Wilson, 1990). At various points during exposure

Table 6.   Different lengths of toxicological study.

Study	Time Scale	Endpoints Commonly Measured
Subacute	Up to 14 days	BAL, biochemistry
Sub-chronic	Up to 90 days	Biochemistry, histopathology, lung burden
Chronic	6 months to 2 years	Biochemistry, histopathology, lung burden
Carcinogenicity	24–30 months	Biochemistry, histopathology, lung burden
Mechanistic	Often short-term	BAL, special techniques, lung burden

and post-exposure, rats are killed for various endpoints. Conventional protocols are shown in Table 6.

Monitoring exposure, dose and response

The key components of the toxicological paradigm, exposure, dose and response, require particular attention in inhalation toxicology, in order to interpret results. The exposure needs to be carried out with a cloud of particles of the correct Dae to ensure sufficient deposition of the material in the area of interest e.g. the airways or the respiratory zone (Schlesinger *et al.*, 1998). The cutoffs for these regions can be very steep in the rat and so this requires due consideration and monitoring. Serial kills of rats need to be carried out for quantification of the lung tissue concentration of the particles to ensure that adequate dosing of the target tissues was achieved. This is usually achieved by ashing or digestion of the lung tissue and mass or chemical measures of the particle burden per lung [e.g. This can be refined with counts of particle sizes e.g. fibres) or preliminary micro-dissection of lung to quantify distribution within different lung compartments (e.g. pleura or alveolar ducts)]. The response can be from the extent of inflammation to the proportion of tumours and is discussed below.

The maximum tolerated dose and overload

As a result of the increasing demonstration and elucidation of the phenomenon of "overload" in laboratory rats exposed to low toxicity dusts, the choice of the exposure regimen is increasingly important.

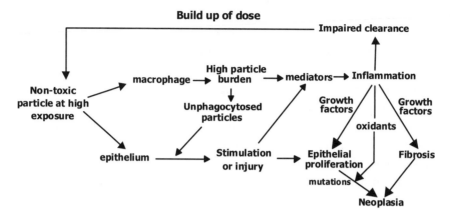

Fig. 4. A hypothetical model for the events during overload.

Classical overload occurs in rats exposed to very high levels of airborne particles, which accumulate in the lungs to a point where there is failure of clearance, increased build-up of dose, inflammation, proliferation, fibrosis and tumour production (Mauderly and McCunney, 1996). The mechanism of overload is not well understood, but the essential elements are shown in Fig. 4.

The important implication for inhalation toxicology is that a sufficiently high enough exposure to any airborne particle will result in a false-positive pathological outcome. The Maximum Tolerated Dose (MTD) is a concept that takes this into account and seeks to carry out the exposure at a level that does not overwhelm the defences or detoxification functions of the target tissue, causing the elicitation of a response that does not occur at plausible exposure levels. The play-off is thus between MTD and increasing the exposure to counteract the relative insensitivity of rat bioassays, which commonly use only up to 50 rats per dose group, whereas most human adverse effects arise at less than 1 in 50 individuals. The MTD is obtained from range-finding studies that seek to determine at which point in the dose scale there is an alteration in the linear nature of the target organ response. Operationally in inhalation toxicology, this means that the MTD exposure concentration is chosen as the maximum exposure at which there is no impairment of clearance, i.e. below the overload level.

To prevent confusion because of an effect of overload in studies with low toxicity particles, the exposure should be carried out at an exposure that does not cause inhibition of clearance or excessive inflammation. The mass of particulate in the lungs does not appear to be the best metric for predicting overload, but surface area does appear to predict onset of overload for two very different no-toxic particles (Tran *et al.*, 1998); the surface area dose that cause overload was 2–300 cm^2 per rat. Thus, dosimetry in terms of surface area as well as mass should also be considered when choosing the exposure concentration and the exposure regimen.

Immunological effects of particles

In the case of particles that may be sensitising or may elicit effects in sensitised individuals, special testing can be carried out. Kimber and co-workers (e.g. Kimber *et al.*, 1996) have published bioassays for detecting respiratory allergens based on two approaches: (1) the conventional detection of IgE against the allergen, (2) lung lymph node cells from animals treated with the respiratory allergen that are tested for Th2 cytokines interleukins 4 and 10 and the Th1 cell cytokine interferon gamma where the former are generally increased in mice exposed to respiratory allergens. These assays can be expected to become more refined as the mechanism of allergic lung disease improves. For particle suspected of causing extrinsic allergic alve-olitis, BAL profile, tests for complement activation and specific IgM and IgG, and histological evidence of granulomatous disease should be carried out following conventional intratracheal or instillation exposure (Sharma and Fujimara, 1995). For particles that might be expected to exacerbate asthma, Gilmour and co-workers (1996) have described assays to assess the effect of co-exposure to pollutants on the immune and inflammatory response to common allergens.

Effects on the microbicidal activity of the lungs

The ability of the lung to resist infection is an important function that could be compromised by exposure to particles, since particles could have effects on macrophages and epithelial cells that could compromise their microbicidal functions. This has been reviewed recently by Thomas and Zelikoff (1999). Impairment of pulmonary defences against bacteria are described, following exposure to metals and to woodsmoke particles. This is an important area where more information is needed and where specific particle might have considerable impact.

3. Conclusion: A Tiered Approach to Testing of a New Particle

The following represents summary of the approach taken here for the testing of the particle of the unknown toxicity. It is a tiered system that can be entered at any point or stopped at any point, giving various degrees of confidence about the potential toxicity:

(1) Consider the size of the particle and draw conclusions about its site of deposition and the likelihood of substantial deposition in the different compartments of the lungs.

(2) Determine the composition and biopersistence of the particle and benchmark the particle against other similarly structured particles to anticipate the likelihood and types of adverse effects.

(3) Armed with the data from benchmarking, carry out appropriate cell tests to determine whether there is any evidence for toxicity.

(4) Carry out instillation studies with due consideration of dose and inclusion of positive and negative control particles.

(5) Carry out inhalation studies in animals, but also potentially in man.

(6) To understand the mechanism of toxic action of particles, further reductionist mechanistic studies on the cellular and molecular responses elicited by the particles can be carried out.

At any point in the above tiered approach, the particle may be exonerated from likely toxic effects and the subsequent testing tiers need not be carried out. Conversely, the system may also illustrate an important aspect of toxicity that deserves further study in specialised protocols.

References

Angel, P. and Karin, M. (1991) The role of Jun, Fos and the AP-1 complex in cell proliferation and transformation. *Biochim Biophys Acta* **1072**: 129–157.

Baker S.J., Kerppola T.K., Luk D., Vandenberg M.T., Marshak D.R., Curran T. and Abate C. (1992) Jun is phosphorylated by several protein kinases at the same sites that are modified in serum stimulated fibroblasts. *Mol Cell Biol* **12**: 4694–4705.

Berridge M.J. (1993) Inositol trisphosphate and calcium signalling. *Nature* **361**: 315–325.

Berridge M.V., Tan A.S., McCoy K.D. and Wang R. (1996) The biochemical and cellular basis of cell proliferation assays that use tetrazolium salts. *Biochemica* **4**: 15–20.

BeruBe K.A., Quinlan T.R., Fung H., Magae J., Vacek P., Taatjes D.J. and Mossman B.T. (1996) Apoptosis is observed in mesothelial cells after exposure to crocidolite asbestos. *Am J Respir Cell Mol Biol* 14

Brown D.M., Beswick P.H. and Donaldson K. (in press) Induction of nuclear translocation of NF-κB in epithelial cells by respirable fibres. *J Pathol.*

Brown D.M. and Donaldson K. (1996) Wool and grain dusts stimulate TNF secretion by alveolar macrophages *in vitro*. *Occup Env Med* **53**: 387–393.

Carter A.B., Monick M.M. and Hunninghake G.W. (1998) Lipopolysaccharide-induced NF-kB activation and cytokine release in human alveolar macrophages is PKC-independent and TK- and PC-PLC-dependent. *Am J Respir Cell Mol Biol* **18**: 384–391.

Carter J.D., Ghio A.J., Samet J.M. and Devlin R.B. (1997) Cytokine production by human airway epithelial cells after exposure to an air pollution particle is metal-dependent. *Toxicol Pharmacol* **146**: 180–188.

Castranova V., Dalal N.S. and Vallyathan V. (1995) The role of surface free radicals in the pathogenicity of silicosis in Silica and silica-induced lung diseases. CRC Press, Boca Raton.

Chabot F., Mitchell J.A., Gutteridge J.M.C. and Evans T.W. (1998) Reactive oxygen species in acute lung injury. *Eur Respir J* **11**: 745–757.

Chen J., Armstrong L.C., Liu S., Gerriets J.E. and Last J.A. (1991) Silica increases cytosolic free calcium ion concentration of alveolar macrophages *in vitro*. *Toxicol Appl Pharmacol* **111**: 211–220.

Chow C.-W., Grinstein S. and Rotstein O.D. (1995) Signaling events in monocytes and macrophages. *New Horizons* **3**(2): 342–351.

Churg A. and Green F.H.Y. (1998) Pathology of Occupational Lung Disease. 2nd Edition.Williams and Wilkins, Baltimore.

Coin P.G., Roggli V.L. and Brody A.R. (1994) Persistence of long, thin chrysotile asbestos fibers in the lungs of rats. *Environ Health Perspect* **102**(Suppl)5: 197–199.

Davis J.M.G., Addison J., Bolton R.E., Donaldson K., Jones A.D. and Smith T. (1986). The pathogenicity of long versus short fibre samples of amosite asbestos administered to rats by inhalation and intraperitoneal injection. *Brit J Exp Pathol* **67**: 415–430.

Davis J.M.G., Brown D.M., Cullen R.T., Donaldson K., Jones A.D., Miller B.G., McIntosh C. and Searl A. (1996) A comparison of methods of determining and predicting the pathogenicity of mineral fibers. *Inhal Toxicol* **8**: 747–770.

Donaldson K., Li X.Y. and MacNee W. (1998) Ultrafine (nanometer) particle-mediated lung injury. *J Aerosol Sci* **29**: 553–560.

Donaldson K. and Borm P. (1998) The quartz hazard: A variable entity. *Ann Occup Hyg* **42**: 287–294.

Donaldson K., Li X.Y. and MacNee W. (1998) Ultrafine (nanometer) particle medi-ated lung injury. *J Aerosol Sci* **29**: 553–560.

Donaldson K. (1998) Mechanisms of pneumoconiosis. in Occupational Lung Dis-ease. An international perspective. Banks DE and Parker JE (eds.). Chapman and Hall Medical. London, pp. 139–160.

Donaldson K. and MacNee W. (1998) The mechanism of lung injury caused by PM_{10}. In Air pollution and Health. *Issues Environ Sci Technol* **10**: 21–32.

Dreher K., Costa D., Jaskot R. and Kodavanti U. (1995) Role of soluble metals in the acute pulmonary toxicity of an emission source particulate. *Faseb J* **9**: A–A.

Driscoll K.E. (1996) Role of inflammation in the development of rat lung tumors in response to chronic particle exposure. *Inhal Toxicol* **8** (suppl): 139–153.

Droge W., Schulzeosthoff K., Mihm S., Galter D., Schenk H., Eck H.P., Roth S. and Gmunder H. (1994) Functions of glutathione and glutathione disulfide immunol-ogy and immunopathology. *Faseb J* **8**: 1131–1138.

Faux S.P., Michelangeli F. and Levy L.S. (1994) Calcium chelator quin-2 prevents crocidolite-induced DNA strand breakage in human white blood cells. *Muta Res* **311**: 209–215.

Faux S.P., Janssen Y.M.W., Torino J., Timblin C.R., Quinlan T.Q., Zanella C.L. and Mossman B.T. Extracellular calcium stimulates both CREB and AP-1 transcription factors and c-fos in rat pleural mesothelial cells following exposure to asbestos. Submitted for publication.

Fubini B. Bolis V., Cavenago A. and Volante M. (1995) Physicochemical proper-ties of crystalline silica dusts and their possible implication in various biological responses. *Scand J Work Environ Health* **21**: 9–14.

Fubini B.A.E.. Aust Bolton R.E., Borm P.J.A., Bruch J., Ciapetti G., Donaldson K., Elias Z., Gold J., Jaurand M.-C., Kane A.B., Lison D. and Muhle H. (1998) Non-animal tests for evaluating the toxicity of solid xenobiotics. *ECVAM Workshop* Report 30. ATLA; **26**: 579–617

Ghio A.J., Jaskot R.H. and Hatch G.E. (1994) Lung injury after silica instillation is associated with an accumulation of iron in rats. *Am J Physiol-Lung Cell Mol Physio* **11**: L-L.

Gilmour P.S., Brown D.M., Beswick P.H., MacNee W., Rahman I. and Donaldson K. (1997) Free radical activity of industrial fibers: Role of iron in oxidative stress and activation of transcription factors. *Environ Health Perspec* **105**(Suppl)5: 1313–1317.

Gilmour P.S., Brown D.M., Lindsay T.G., Beswick P.H., MacNee W. and Donaldson K. (1996) Adverse health effects of PM$_{10}$: Involvement of iron in the generation of hydroxyl radical. *Occupat Environ Med* **53**: 817–822.

Gilmour M.I., Park P. and Selgrade M.J. (1996) Increased immune and inflammatory responses to dust mite antigen in rats exposed to 5 ppm NO2. *Fundamental Appl Toxicol* **31**: 65–70.

Grynkiewicz G., Poenie M. and Tsein R.Y. (1985) A new generation of Ca2+ indicators with greatly improved fluorescent properties. *J Biol Chem* **260**(6): 3440–3450.

Guthrie G.D. and Heath C.W. (1995) Mineralogical charcteristics of silica polymorphs in relatoin to their biological activities. Anonymous. *Scand J Work Environ Health* **21**(Suppl 2): 5–8.

Heintz N.H., Janssen Y.M.W. and Mossman B.T. (1993) Persistent induction of c-fos and c-jun expression by asbestos. *Proc Natl Acad Sci USA* **90**: 3299–3303.

Henderson R.F., Driscoll K.E., Harkema J.R., Lindenschmidt R.C., Chang I.Y., Maples K.R. and Barr E.B. (1995) A comparison of the inflammatory response of the lung to inhaled versus instilled particles in f344 rats. *Fund Appl Toxicol* **24**: 183–197.

Hesterberg T.W., Miiller W.C., Mast R., Mcconnell E.E., Bernstein D.M. and Anderson R. (1994) Relationship between lung biopersistence and biological effects of man-made vitreous fibers after chronic inhalation in rats. *Environ Health Perspect* **102**: 133–137.

Howden P.J. and Faux S.P. (1997) Possible role of lipid peroxidation in the induction of NF-kB and AP-1 in RFL-6 cells by crocidolite asbestos: Evidence following protection by vitamin E. *Environ Health Perspect* **105**: 1127–1130.

International Standards Organisation. (1994) Air quality: Particle size fraction definitions for health-related sampling. IS 7708, ISO, Geneva.

Isreal A. (1995) A role for phosphorylation and degradation in the control of NF-κB activity. *Trends Genet* **11**: 203–205.

Iyer R., Hamilton R.F., Li L. and Holian A. (1996) Silica-induced apoptosis mediated via scavenger receptor in human alveolar macrophages. *Toxicol Appl Pharmacol* **140**:

Janknecht R., Cahill M.A. and Nordheim A. (1995) Signal transduction at the c-fos promotor. *Carcinogenesis* **16**: 443–450.

Janssen Y.M., Barchowsky A., Treadwell M., Driscoll K.E. and Mossman B.T. (1995) Asbestos induces nuclear factor κB (NF-κB) DNA-binding activity and NF-κB dependent gene expression in tracheal epithelial cells. *Proc Natl Acad Sci USA* **92**: 8458–8462.

Kamp D.W., Graceffa P., Pryor W.A. and Weitzman S.A. (1992) The role of free radicals in asbestos-induced diseases. *Free Rad Biol Med* **12**(4): 293–315.

Karin M. (1995) The regulation of AP-1 by mitogen-activated protein kinases. *J Biol Chem* **270**: 16483–16486.

Kennedy T.P., Dodson R., Rao N.V., Ky H., Hopkins C., Baser M., Tolley E. and Hoidal J.R. (1989) Dusts causing pneumoconiosis generate oh and produce hemolysis by acting as fenton catalysts. *Arch Biochem Biophy* **269**: 359–364.

Kimber I., Hilton J., Basketter D.A. and Dearman R.J. (1996) Predictive testing for respiratory sensitization in the mouse. *Toxicol Lett* **86**: 193–198.

Kodavanti U.P., Jaskot R.H., Costa D.L. and Dreher K.L. (1997) Pulmonary proin-flammatory gene induction following acute exposure to residual oil fly ash: Roles of particle-associated metals. *Inhal Toxicol* **9**: 679–701.

Korzeniewski C. and Callewaert D.M. (1983) An enzyme-release assay for natural cytotoxicity. *J Immunol Meth* **64**: 313–320.

LaRosa F.A., Pierce J.W. and Sonenshein G.E. (1994) Differential regulation of the c-myc oncogene promoter by the NF-κB rel family of transcription factors. *Mol Cell Biol* **14**: 1039–1044.

Lim Y., Kim S.-H., Cho Y.-J., Kim K.-A., Oh M.-W. and Lee K.-H. (1997) Silica induced oxygen radical generation in alveolar macrophage. *Ind Health* **35**: 380–387.

Liu R.-M., Hu H., Robinson T.W. and Forman H.J. (1996) Differential enhance-ment of g-glutamyl transpeptidase and g-glutamylcysteine synthetase by tert-butylhydroquinone in rat lung epithelial L2 cells. *Am J Respir Cell Mol Biol* **14**: 186–191.

Lund L.G. and Aust E. (1992) Iron mobilization from crocidolite asbestos greatly enhances crocidolite-dependent formation of DNA single-strand breaks in ϕX174 RFI DNA. *Carcinogenesis* **13**: 637–642.

Maltoni C., Minardi F. and Morisi L. (1982) Pleural mesotheliomas in Sprague-Dawley rats by erionite: First experimental evidence. *Environ Res* **29**(1): 238–244,

Mauderly J.L. and McCunney R.J. (1996) Particle overload in the rat lung: Implications for human risk assessment. Anonymous. Anonymous. *Inhal Toxicol* **8**(Suppl): 298.

McConkey D.J. and Orrenius S. (1997) The role of calcium in the regulation of apoptosis. *Biochem Biophys Res Commun* **239**: 357–366.

Melloni B., Lesur O., T. Bouhadiba T., Cantin A., Martel M. and Begin R. (1996) Effect of exposure to silica on human alveolar macrophages in supporting growth activity in type II epithelial cells. *Thorax* **51**: 781–786.

Meyer M., Schreck R. and Baeuerle P.A. (1993) H2O2 and antioxidant have oppo-site effects on activation of NF-kB and AP-1 in intact cells: AP-1 as a secondary antioxidant-response factor. *EMBO J* **12**: 2005–2015.

Morgan W.K.C. and Seaton A. (1995) *Occupational Lung Diseases*. Saunders, Philadelphia.

Mossmann T. (1983) Rapid colorimetric assay for cellular growth and survival: Appli-cation to proliferation and cytotoxicity assays. *J Immunol Meth* **65**: 55–63.

Oberdorster G. (1995) Lung particle overload: Implications for occupational expo-sure to particles. *Reg Toxicol Pharmacol* **27**: 123–135.

Palombella V.J., Rando O.J., Goldberg A.L. and Maniatis T. (1994) The ubiquitin-proteosome pathway is required for processing the NF-κB1 precursor protein and the activation of NF-κB. Cell **78**: 773–785.

Parkes W.R. (1994) *Occupational Lung Disorders.* Butterworth-Heinemann.

Parekh A.B. and Penner R. (1997) Store depletion and calcium influx. *Physiol Rev* **77**(4): 901–930.

Peces R. and Urra J.M. (1995) Effect of calcium-channel blocker on tumour necrosis factor alpha (TNFα) production in cyclosporin-treated renal transplant recipients. *Nephrol Dial Transplant* **10**: 871–873.

Peters A., Wichmann H.E., Tuch T., Heinrich J. and Heyder J. Respiratory effects are associated with the number of ultrafine particles. *Am J Respir Crit Care Med* **155**: 1376–1383, 1997.

Quay J.L, Reed W., Samet J. and Devlin R.B. (1998) Air pollution particles induce IL-6 gene expression in human airway epithelial cells via NF-kB activation. *Am J Respir Cell Mol Biol* **19**: 98–106.

Rahman I. and MacNee W. (1998) Role of transcription factors in inflammatory lung diseases. *Thorax* **53**: 601–612.

Rahman I., Bel A., Mulier B., Lawson M.F., Harrison D.J., MacNee W. and Smith C.A.D. (1996) Transcriptional regulation of γ-glutamylcysteine sythetase-heavy subunit by oxidants in human alveolar epithelial cells. Biochemical and Biophysical Research Communications **229**: 832–837.

Schins *et al.*

Schlesinger R.B., Bender J.R., Dahl A.R., Snipes M.B. and Ultman J. (1998) Deposition of inhaled toxicicants, in *Handbook of Human Toxicology.* Massaro EJ (ed.).CRC Press, Boca Raton, pp. 493–550.

Schmitz R. and Baeuerle P. (1991) The p65 subunit is responsible for the strong transcription activating potential of NF-κB. EMBO J. **10**: 3805–3817.

Schwartz J., Dockery D.W. and Neas L.M. (1996) Is daily mortality associated specifically with fine particles. *J Air Waste Manag Assoc* **46**: 927–939.

Seaton A., MacNee W., Donaldson K. and Godden D. (1995) Particulate air pollution and acute health effects. *Lancet* **345**: 176–178.

Seger R. and Krebbs E.G. (1995) The MAPK signalling cascade. *FASEB J* **9**: 726–735.

Sen C.K. and Packer L. (1996) Antioxidant and redox regulation of gene transcription. *FASEB J* **10**: 709–720.

Simeonova P.P. and Luster M.I. (1996) Asbestos induction of nuclear transcription factors and interleukin 8 gene regulation. *Am J Respir Cell Mol Biol* **15**: 787–795.

Stanton M.F., Layard M., Tegeris A., Miller E., May M., Morgan E. and Smith A. (1981) Relation of particle dimension to carcinogenicity in amphibole asbestoses and other fibrous minerals. *J Nat Cancer Inst* **67**(5): 965–975.

Stone V., Shaw J., Brown D.M., MacNee W., Faux S.P. and Donaldson K. (1998) The role of oxidative stress in the prolonged inhibitory effect of ultrafine carbon black on epithelial cell function. *Toxicol In Vitro* **12**: 649–659.

Stone V., Tuinman M., Vamvakopoulos J.E., Faux S.P., Borm P., MacNee W. and Donaldson K. Increased calcium influx on exposure to ultrafine carbon black: A potential mechanism for the pathogenicity of ultrafine particles.

Thanos D. and Maniatis T. (1995) NF-kB: A lesson in family values. *Cell* **80**: 529–532.

Thastrup O., Cullen P.J., Drobak B.K., Hanley M.R. and Dawson A.P. (1990) Thapsigargin, a tumour promoter, discharges intracellular Ca2+ stores by specific inhibition of the endoplasmic reticulum Ca2+-ATPase. *Proc Natl Acad Sci USA* **87**: 2466–2470.

Thomas P.T. and Zelikoff J.T. (1999) Air pollutants: Modulators of pulmonary host resistance against infection in Air pollution and health. ST Holgate, JM Samet, HS Koren,RL Maynard (eds.). Academic Press, London, 357–379.

Timblin C.R., Janssen Y.W.M. and Mossman B.T. (1995) Transcriptional activation of the proto-oncogene c-jun by asbestos and H2O2 is directly related to increased proliferation and transformation of tracheal epithelial cells. *Cancer Res* **55**: 2723–2726.

Timblin C.R., BeruBe K.A., Churg A., Driscoll K.E, Gordon T., Hemenway D., Walsh E., Cummins A.B., Vacek P. and Mossman B.T. (1998) Ambient particulate matter causes activation of the c-jun kinase/stress-activated protein kinase cascade and DNA synthesis in lung epithelial cells. *Cancer Res.* **58**: 4543–4547.

Tran C.L., Jones A.D., Cullen R.T. and Donaldson K. (1998) Influence of particle characteristics on the clearance of low toxicity dusts from the lungs. *J Aerosol Sci* **29**(Suppl 1): S1269–S1270

Warheit D.B, Mchugh T.A., Kellar K.A. and Hartsky M.A. (1993) The low durability of inhaled wollastonite or kevlar(R) Fibers in the lungs of rats correlates with transient pulmonary inflammatory effects. *Am Rev Respir Dis* **147**: A-A.

Wilson A.B.(1990) Experimental design, in *Experimental Toxicology*. Royal Society of Chemistry, The Universities Press, Belfast, pp. 35–55

Xia Z., Dickens M., Raingeaud J., Davis R.J. and Greenberg M.E. (1995) Opposing effects of ERK and JNK-p38 MAP kinases on apoptosis. *Science* **270**: 1326–1331.

Xie Q.-W., Kashiwabara Y. and Nathan C. (1994) Role of the transcription fator NF-κB/Rel in induction of nitric oxide synthase. *J Biol Chem* **269**: 4705–4708.

CHAPTER 7

VALUING THE HEALTH IMPACT OF AIR POLLUTION: DEATHS, DALYS OR DOLLARS?

A.E.M. de Hollander and J.M. Melse

1. Fifty Years on

Fifty years after the infamous London smog of 1952 which killed 4,000 to 12,000 inhabitants, air pollution might still be a significant health risk factor (Ministry of Health, 1954; Bell and Davis, 2001). Since those days, air pollution in Western Europe has changed greatly with regard to both composition and concentrations. In the 19th century, despite some legislation to prevent smoke nuisance from industrial emissions, levels of fossil fuel-related pollutants, such as smoke and sulphur dioxide, were at least tenfold higher than nowadays. Up to the 1960s, in major cities such as London, Paris or Amsterdam, the bulk of air pollution came from domestic sources, since the widespread use of coal, especially for domestic fire has almost completely disappeared. High sulphur coal of varying quality was replaced by natural gas of which abundant stocks were discovered in the 60s, e.g. in the North Sea and north-eastern parts of the Netherlands. However, in the same period, road traffic volume grew exponentially and in spite of impressive, concurrent development of clean engine technology, road traffic is now the most important source of air pollution, accounting for more than one third of fine particulate matter (PM_{10})

emissions (for the smaller fractions, $PM_{2.5}$, more than half) and more than half of nitrogen dioxide emissions.

It is generally accepted that till today, ambient air pollution still affects public health, although the precise causal fraction of the air pollutant mix remains a subject of fierce debate (Brunekreef, 1999; Brunekreef and Holgate, 2002). As we spend the greater part of our days inside houses and buildings, indoor air pollution is inevitably of great relevance to public health as well, in particular, exposure to radon, second hand tobacco smoke and dampness-related allergens, all of which contribute significantly to disease burden (de Hollander *et al.*, 1999). In most Western European countries, environmental policy is not very much concerned with indoor air quality, at least not in the light of recent discussions on (proposed) legislation with respect to ambient air pollution. Nevertheless, in this chapter, health impacts of indoor air pollution will be considered as a reference to put the ambient air pollution health risk debate in a wider perspective.

2. Problems for Policy Makers

The rapid advancements in statistical methodology have not really made life easier for policy makers involved in air pollution control. In the "good old days", risk managers would judge the air quality by compliance with health-based standards. As long as concentrations of air pollutants were below these standards the air was "safe" to breathe. Whenever concentrations started to exceed standards regularly, public health was at stake and risk-reducing measures had to be considered. These standards were and still are often primarily based on guidelines derived by expert committees after careful consideration of available toxicological and epidemiological evidence. These "compound by compound" evaluations are completed with proposals for safe ambient air pollution concentrations using simple, quantitative models. In these models, science, societal preferences and policy are elegantly mixed, as establishing air quality guidelines requires several normative choices to be made (World Health Organization, 2000; Health Council of the Netherlands, 1996). For instance, one has to define critical toxicological end-points and decide on the extent of the safety margins, given the quantity and quality of the exposure-response data.

Current epidemiological insights do not comply very well with this type of quality standard-based risk management, as clear evidence of a threshold for the health end-points considered appears to be lacking, at least at realistic levels of ambient air pollutant concentrations (Brunekreef and Holgate, 2002). Furthermore, the observed end-points include a large variety of health effects, ranging from mild, reversible lung function deficits, slightly restricted potential for physical activity to hospital admission and mortality among the susceptible (Fig. 1). Obviously the nature, frequency and severity of the health effects depend largely on the individual's health status. In this situation, drawing the line between trivial and health threatening responses is difficult.

In the absence of clearly defined safe or virtually safe levels, there is no easy way out of discussions on the acceptability of health

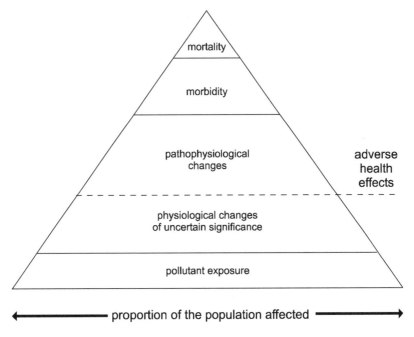

Fig. 1. Schematic representation of the distribution of air pollution responses in the population.

responses associated with population exposure to air pollution. In the last few decades, much effort has been put into controlling air pollution, associated with key activities such as transport, energy production, industry, and waste treatment. Current levels are largely determined by best available technology and further emission reductions to meet more stringent standards would require ever-bigger resources. Beside constraints on the opportunities for economic activity that might produce more wealth and well being, these resources cannot be used for other things we value, such as health care or the quality of the urban environment. Furthermore, several analyses have cast some doubt on the efficiency of standard-based health risk management, as very expensive measures often appear to yield fairly minor public health gains (and vice versa) (Tengs *et al.*, 1995). Some authors even suggest that very expensive life-saving regulations might be counterproductive, as a drop in the aggregate national income of approximately EUR 8 million will theoretically induce one extra fatality (Gerdtham and Johannesson, 2002). Table 1 shows a remarkable variation in costs per healthy life-year that is saved for a broad range of life saving interventions, of which environmental measures are often found at the more expensive end of the distribution (de Hollander, 2003).

3. Putting Money where Public Health Profits Most

As pure standard-based decision rules no longer seem to apply fully, a shift is occurring towards rules based on "utility", putting the money where public health profits most (Morgan, 1993). This is not without significance as environmental quality standards traditionally stand for *equity*, the right to protection from adverse effects for everybody, regardless of age, health, and susceptibility (right-based decision rules). On the other hand, from an utilitarian perspective, maximisation of utility (efficiency) may require a more skewed distribution of health risk over societal groups, simply because it would be more cost-effective. In other words, guaranteeing the last citizen in town the general level of health protection can be extremely expensive (Morgan, 2000). According to neo-classical economic theory, the trade-off between efficiency and equity becomes an issue (Hammitt, 2002).

Table 1.   Overview of cost-effectiveness calculations for a series of interventions in different population health status domains.

Costs: Euro/QALYa	Intervention
< 0 (cost-saving)	National vaccination programme (DP)b PKU test, neonatal heel prick (DP) Screening of pregnant women for syphilis (DP) Influenza vaccination for chronically ill elderly people (DP) Smoke detector in the home (HPt) Help with addiction to smoking (HP) Removal of lead from petrol and paint, stripping lead-based paint coats (HPt)
0–1,000	Mandatory safety belt (HPt) Disease coping training for asthma (MC) Screening and treatment of chlamydia (DP) Practical test for moped and autocycle (low-speed moped) riders (HPt)
1,000–10,000	Chlorination of drinking water (HPt) Specific vaccinations, e.g. meningococcus C (DP) Treatment of mild to moderate hypertension with beta blockers and anti-diuretics (DP) HIV screening of visitors to sexually transmitted disease (STD) clinics (DP) Influenza vaccination for all elderly people (DP) Cholesterol test and dietary advice (DP) Bypass operation (MC) Stroke units (MC) Viagra (MC) Mammography population survey (DP)
10,000–100,000	Heart transplant (MC) Controlling Legionella in (health) care facilities (HPt) Pneumococcal vaccination for the elderly (DP) Kidney replacing treatments (dialysis) (MC) Smear and treatment for cervical cancer (DP) Periodic automobile test (HPt) Treatment for mild to moderate hypertension with ACE inhibitors, etc. (DP) Airbags (HPt) Ban on asbestos in brake blocks (HPt) Helicopter trauma team (MC) Lung transplant (MC)
100,000–1,000,000	Reduction of radon in existing dwellings (HPt) Neurosurgery for malignant brain tumours (MC) EPO for anaemia in renal dialysis patients (MC) General measures for controlling Legionella in water distribution systems (HPt)
> 1,000,000	Measures for reducing industrial benzene emission in the USA (HPt) Measure to reduce dioxin emissions from waste incinerators (HPt) General measures to reduce exposure to ELF associated with electric power lines (HPt) Earthquake-proof dwellings in parts of the USA (HPt)

aQALY: quality-adjusted life-year.
bDP: disease prevention, HPt: health protection, HP: health promotion, MC: medical care.

From a utilitarian perspective, when considering air pollution, certain questions have to be addressed:

(1) How bad is this environmental exposure, e.g. compared with other environmental exposures or to other health risks in general?
(2) How does public health benefit from policy measures to reduce public exposure?
(3) What policy measures are most efficient or what is the optimal deployment of available resources in terms of health gains?

To describe and compare the health impact of various environmental exposures, and eventually to perform cost effectiveness analysis of options for environmental policies, some sort of "denominator" is obviously required. In general, three ways of characterising potential health benefits are being used, i.e. health risk reduction (numbers), (health adjusted) life-years (e.g. quality adjusted life years — QALYs — or disability adjusted life years — DALYs) or money ("monetarised" health endpoints) (Hofstetter and Hammitt, 2002).

3.1. *Numbers*

To characterise the health impact of air pollution or any other risk factor, one can simply calculate the number of cases of health damage associated with a certain exposure distribution, such as deaths, hospital admissions or number of asthma attacks. In traditional quantitative risk analysis, health risks are measured and often implicitly compared in terms of annual mortality risk: numbers per year. In several Western countries, environmental regulation with respect to industrial safety, radiation protection or chemical pollutants is based on a small "accepted" annual mortality risk for each exposed individual. Often, an individual risk criterion in the order of 10^{-5} or 10^{-6} is used as a threshold of acceptability (Ministry of Housing, 1989; World Health Organization, 1987; National Research Council, 1983). Such an approach guarantees that everybody is at least treated in the same way, whether they are young or old, rich or poor; it prevents inequity as a result of "unloading" health risk on smaller groups of individuals, which is often the low-cost solution (Morgan, 2000).

3.2. *Health Adjusted Life-Years (e.g. DALYs)*

However, it has become clear that one "annual ten to the minus six" risk may differ substantially from another in several important aspects (Health Council of the Netherlands, 1996), such as loss of *life expectancy* and *non-lethal health outcomes*. For instance, mortality during particulate air pollution episodes may, at least in part, involve "precipitation" of death among the old and weak, thus costing several months of unhealthy life at the most (Vedal, 1997; Brunekreef, 1997; Ad-Hoc group, 1999), while the impact associated with fatal accidents in individuals with a "random" age distribution may amount to a loss of many healthy years (Ten Berge and Stallen, 1995). In addition, public health focus has gradually changed from life expectancy to health expectancy, i.e. postponing as long as possible or mitigating the functional limitations that come with chronic disease of older age and that affect the ability to cope with the demands of daily life (World Bank, 1993; Ruwaard and Kramers, 1998). This applies similarly to the health impact of air pollution. In many cases, these do not involve mortality, often not even morbidity, but rather aspects of the quality of life, such as:

(1) Aggravation of pre-existing disease symptoms, e.g. asthma, chronic bronchitis, cardiovascular or psychological disorders.
(2) Severe annoyance, sleep disturbance, reduced ability to concentrate, communicate or perform normal daily tasks.
(3) Feelings of insecurity or alienation, unfavourable health perception and stress in relation to poor quality of the local environment and perceived danger of large fatal accidents (de Hollander and Staatsen, 2003).

Thus, mortality risk is often not the most appropriate indicator of environmental risk.

In an utilitarian approach to maximising cost-effectiveness for society, one would want to employ some sort of public health currency unit representing the full attributable health loss. Over the last few years, much effort has been put into the development of metrics in which any type of morbidity or mortality is transformed into an equivalent number of life years (quantity plus quality of life).

This type of health aggregating metric allows formal analysis of cost-effectiveness of environmental policy measures, which has by now become a rather common practice in medical technology assessment and public health research (World Bank, 1993; Saltman and Figueras, 1997; Hofstetter and Hammitt, 2002).

3.3. Monetary Value

Alongside the cost-effectiveness analysis, cost-benefit analysis is a form of evaluation in which the (health) benefits are also expressed in monetary terms. Efficiency calculations are made easier by putting cost and benefits under one heading, namely money. Furthermore, it is easier to include non-health aspects on the benefit side (equity, productivity, well-being). In principle, investments in the health domain can be compared with investments outside, for instance, transport safety, education, or ecological quality. Obviously, this form of analysis means expressing loss of life, life-years, or the burden of disease in monetary terms, which is a difficult task. In such a "hardcore" economic approach, one seeks to attach a price tag to the incidence of different health end-points, e.g. by investigating people's willingness to pay (WTP) to prevent defined health endpoints, or the amount of money for which people are willing to accept (WTA) a certain level of health risk. In some studies, the costs of productivity loss and health care use are primarily estimated (Krupnick and Portney, 1991; Ostro and Chestnut, 1998; Aunan et al., 1998; USEPA, 1996; Holland et al., 1998). Of course, the latter approach would not include the price of individual suffering.

In this chapter, we investigate the feasibility of paradigms of risk management (mortality risk, numbers), attributable burden of disease (DALYs) and monetary economic evaluation to support public health policy with respect to air pollution. We will focus on the health loss associated with the major air pollution phenomena in the Netherlands (indoor as well as outdoor). Our calculations are based on health impact estimates for the Dutch population, which were produced in the framework of the fourth National Environmental Outlook (National Institute of Public Health and the Environment, 2000).

4. Healthy Time as a Metric

Accepting the fact that annual mortality or even loss of life expectancy do not fully represent the environmental health loss, we have applied an approach largely based on the "burden of disease" measure developed by Murray and Lopez, who used DALYs to assess the global disease burden and consequently the health policy priorities in different regions in the world. This health impact measure combines years of life lost and years lived with disability that are standardised by means of severity weights (World Bank, 1993; Murray and Lopez, 1996). Our adaptation of the DALY concept was inspired by the notion that the multiform health loss due to environmental exposure is fairly well characterised by three dominant aspects of public health:

(1) *Quantity* of life (life expectancy).
(2) *Quality* of life.
(3) *Social magnitude* (or number of people affected).

The diagram in Fig. 2 sketches the basic idea behind our approach. At birth, each of us may expect an approximate potential of eighty years of healthy life. However, due to our genetic programming, our often-unfavourable life-styles, poverty, occupational or environmental conditions, or just misfortune, most of us will encounter diseases that will reduce the quality of part of our life-years. These diseases may manifest themselves in episodes, such as chronic disease or even progressive disability until death. Some of us will die abruptly, for instance, caused by an accident or an infectious disease. Thus, public health loss is defined as time spent with reduced quality of life, aggregated over the population involved. Based on this concept, health loss attributable to air pollution can be assessed by:

(1) Defining responses that are associated with air pollution exposure.
(2) Calculating the number of people affected (N).
(3) Estimating the average duration of the response (including loss of life expectancy as a consequence of premature mortality, D).
(4) Attributing disability weights to each unfavourable health condition (Box 1 & Fig. 3).

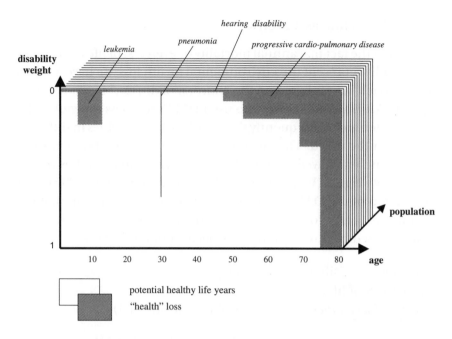

Fig. 2. The concept of disability adjusted life-years.

Finally, we estimate the number of disability adjusted life years that is lost per year of exposure, using the following equation:

$$DALY_{e.e.} = \sum_{i=1}^{n} \sum_{k} I_k * f_k(RR_i, C_i) * S_k * D_k, \quad \text{in which}$$

$DALY_{e.e.}$ = health loss related to n environmental exposures, measured as disability or quality adjusted life-years per year of exposure, $f_k(RR_i, C_i)$ = a set of functions (including exposure C_i and associated relative risk measures RR_i) representing the population attributable fraction (PAF) of condition k, I_k = annual incidence of response variable (baseline risk) k, S_k = severity factor discounting time spent with the condition (see previous paragraph, D_k = duration of the condition; in the case of premature mortality: loss of life expectancy.

Box 1. *Severity weights for disease states.*

In the framework of the National Public health Status and Forecast Reports, an estimate was produced of the burden of disease within the Dutch population (Ruwaard and Kramers, 1998). To define "Dutch" severity weights, Stouthard *et al.* selected 55 diagnoses of greatest public health significance in terms of number of patients, and years of (healthy) life lost. These diagnoses were divided in 176 health states of various severity (or disease stage) (Stouthard *et al.*, 1997).

According to the protocol designed by Murray *et al.* (1996), physicians with ample clinical experience were invited to perform the weighting procedures which consisted of two steps. At first, they evaluated a selection of 16 representative indicator states, using two varieties of a person-trade-off approach. This first step of the valuation process was performed during workshops, as deliberation is an explicit part of the protocol. A visual analogue scale (VAS) was added as another instrument of valuation, mainly for the purpose of validation. Furthermore, a standardised classification of the indicator states according to EuroQol-5D+ was provided to assist panel members (Essink-Bot, 1995). This classification instrument involves a three-point scale for six health dimensions, viz. mobility, self-care, daily activities, pain/discomfort, anxiety/depression and cognitive functions. Using the indicator states for "calibration", the remaining health states were valued individually by means of interpolation (ranking health states similar to one or in between two consecutive indicator conditions, Fig. 3).

For air pollution exposure-related chronic disease morbidity for which different health states have been defined, such as asthma or ischaemic heart disease, a severity factor was composed as a prevalence-weighted average, assuming that the environmental exposure had no effect on disease prognoses (Melse and Kramers, 1999) (e.g. mild, moderate and severe asthma). In some cases, weights referred to transition from one severity state to another, for instance, from mild to severe asthma ("aggravation of asthma").

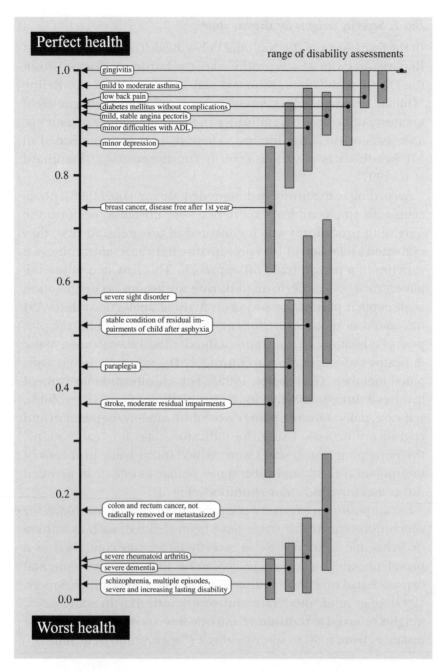

Fig. 3.   Scale of "calibration" health states, employed to attribute weights to health states associated with environmental exposures.

To estimate the number of people affected, we calculated PAFs by combining population exposure distributions with quantitative exposure-response information, applying the following equation (or one its derivatives):

$$PAF = \frac{\sum_{i>0} (RR_i - 1) * p_i}{\sum_{i\geq0} RR_i * p_i},$$

in which RR_i = relative risk in exposure class i and p_i = exposure probability in class i.

Subsequently, we estimated the number of people affected by a certain response by multiplying the PAF with annual incidence figures, obtained from Dutch health statistics, primary care registrations or specific surveys.

5. Trading Health for Wealth or Wealth for Health

While DALYs measure health loss in units of time, applying the WTP (or WTA) approach is an effort to measure health loss in terms of money. Embedded in welfare economics, it should be seen as the rate of substitution between health and wealth. Health is regarded as an economic good. An individual's preference for ones health condition over a certain period of time can be represented by a change of income or wealth, or in other words, decreased possibilities to purchase other valued goods (Hammitt and QALYs versus, 2002). There are two broad ways to produce these estimates:

(1) Investigating how health risks that are related to certain risky occupations are allowed for in the differences in salary, or what extra amount people are prepared to pay for safer or healthier products (e.g. cars with airbags, or houses in quieter surroundings).
(2) Using questionnaires to find out what people are prepared to pay for one extra life-year or one year free of disease or disabilities (contingency valuation).

Significant methodological objections are attached to both methods in connection with the transferability of implicit (behaviour) or explicit (survey) preferences of people from one circumstance to another, including a series of shortcomings that are characteristic of all questionnaire-based surveys (Diener *et al.*, 1998; Klose, 1999; Olsen and Smith, 2001). In terms of the value of a statistical life, the outcomes of the above-mentioned methods are nevertheless reasonably consistent. On average, Americans, Canadians or Europeans are willing to pay in the order of EUR two million for a statistical life (1.5 to 7 million Euros), approximately EUR 70,000 to 80,000 a year at a discount rate of 3% (which is considerably more than an individual's earning capacity, another commonly used proxy) (Melse and de Hollander, 2001; Davis *et al.*, 2002).

6. Impact Assessment

6.1. *Health Responses to Exposures*

Tables 1, 2 and 3 present an overview of the population exposure-response functions for each air pollution type observed in a range of environmental and occupational epidemiological analyses. The associations for fine particulate matter (Table 2) and ozone (Table 3) are presented as increases in end-point incidence per 10 and $150\,\mu g/m^3$ increase of the pollutant concentration, respectively, either based on results of valid Dutch studies or simple random effects meta-analysis (Hollander *et al.*, 1998; Department of Health, 1998).

In all tables, an estimate is given of either incidence (including mortality) or prevalence of the health end-points in the Netherlands. These were based on available Dutch health statistics, summarised in the framework of the National Public Health Status and Forecast Report (Ruwaard and Kramers, 1997, 1998).

Population-weighted exposure distributions for ozone and particles were derived through linear interpolation of data from stationary air pollution monitors of the national network (1997). As urban concentrations of particles tend to be higher, adjustments were made based on the virtual diameter of the urban agglomerations (> 40.000 inhabitants), employing an empirically determined factor. Subsequently, the spatial distribution of air pollutant concentrations was combined with data on population density by means of Geographic

Table 2. Exposure response functions for health effects associated with particulate air pollution.

Health Response (*particulate matter, PM$_{10}$*)	Study Design	Effect Estimate (% per 10 μg/m^3)	Inc/Prev
Long term mortality	Cohort (Dockery *et al.*, 1993; Pope III *et al.*, 1995; Hoek *et al.*, 2002)		
Overall annual mortality		2.4 (0.1–6.1)[a]	0.0078
Cardiopulmonary		4.3 (0.5–11.0)[a]	0.0032
Lung cancer			0.00054
		2.0 (−4.5–8.1)	
Chronic respiratory disease			
Chronic respiratory symptoms in children	Cohort (Dockery *et al.*, 1989; Künzli *et al.*, 2000)	8.7 (0.7–16.6)	0.057
Chronic bronchitis adults	Cohort (Abbey *et al.*, 1991, 1993, 1995; Schwartz, 1993; Aunan, 1996)	2.5 (1.2–3.8)	0.018
Daily mortality	Time series (Hoek *et al.*, 1997)		
Total		0.36 (0.25–0.47)	0.000024
Respiratory disease (COPD)		1.11 (0.64–1.61)	0.00000011
Cardiovascular		0.25 (−0.09–0.42)	0.0000071
Pneumonia			0.00000065
		1.21 (0.65–1.80)	
Hospital admission	Time series		
Respiratory		0.8 (0.5–1.1)	0.0000195
Cardio-vascular		0.7 (0.5–0.9)	0.0000384
Emergency room visits	Time series		
Respiratory		1.5 (0.5–2.6)	0.022
Aggravation of asthma	Panel Studies (Dockery and Pope III, 1994; Roemer *et al.*, 1993; Hoek and Brunekreef, 1994; Hoek and Brunekreef, 1993)		
Attacks		4.4 (−2.0–10.5)	0.00023
Use of bronchodilators		7.0 (0.64–12.9)	0.00059
Respiratory symptoms	Panel studies		
Upper respiratory tract		2.0 (−0.13–4.1)	0.19
Lower respiratory tract		3.8 (0.3–7.1)	0.038

[a]calculated for the fraction highly exposed living within 50, respectively 100 meters distance from a major inner-city road or a freeway, roughly comparable with a concentration difference of 10 μg/m^3 for black smoke, 30 μg/m^3 for NO$_2$ and 40 μg/m^3 for PM$_{10}$ (Brunekree, 1999; Hoek *et al.*, 2002).

Table 3.   Exposure response functions for health effects associated with ozone air pollution.

Health Response Ozone	Study Design	Effect Estimate (% per 150 μg/m³ 8h average)	Inc/Prev
Daily mortality	Time series (Ministry of Health, 1954)		
Total		4.1 (2.0–5.9)	0.000024
Respiratory disease		12.7 (4.8–21.1)	0.00000011
Cardiovascular		3.2 (0.3–6.1)	0.0000071
Pneumonia		18.8 (9.0–29.9)	0.00000065
Hospital admission	Time series (World Bank, 1993)		
Respiratory		6.5 (3.9–9.1)	0.0000195
Emergency room visits	Time series (World Bank, 1993)		
Respiratory		9.1 (2.9–13.8)	0.035

Information Systems (Laboratory for Air Pollution Research, 2003; Eerens *et al.*, 1993).

We recognise the fact that this type of exposure characterisation only poorly reflects personal exposure, which is a function of time-activity patterns and micro-environmental concentrations. On the other hand, epidemiological studies incorporate the same kind of relatively poorly defined ambient air pollution data. Furthermore, at least with respect to particles, a fairly consistent correlation has been shown between ambient and personal exposure indicators (Janssen *et al.*, 1998).

The prevalence of exposure to spousal environmental tobacco smoke was based on cross-sectional monitoring data (Dutch Foundation on Smoking and Health, 1998), assuming that smokers had a risk of living with a smoker three times as high as a non-smoker. Prevalence of damp homes was based on an investigation by the

Table 4.   Exposure response functions for health effects associated with selected air pollutants.

Air Pollutant	Health End-point	Effect Estimate	P_0
Damp houses	Asthma symptoms children	RR_{expo}: 1.41 (1.23–1.71)	0.135
	Asthma prevalence adults	RR_{expo}: 1.56 (1.25–1.95)	0.012
ETS	Lung cancer ns men	RR_{expo}: 1.34 (1.00–1.84)	0.000016
	Lung cancer ns women	RR_{expo}: 1.24 (1.13–1.36)	0.00000074
	IHD nonsmoking men	RR_{expo}: 1.23 (1.03–1.47)	0.0006
	IHD nonsmoking women	RR_{expo}: 1.19 (0.97–1.45)	0.0005
	Aggravation of asthma	RR_{expo}: 1.63 (1.30–1.96)	0.004
	Lower respiratory symptoms	RR_{expo}: 1.46 (1.33–1.60)	0.037
	Otitis media	RR_{expo}: 1.29 (1.05–1.35)	0.00012
	Sudden infant death	RR_{expo}: 1.94 (1.55–2.43)	0.0000037

Table 5.   Exposure distributions for air pollution types.

Air Pollutant	Metric	Mean (stDev)
PM_{10}	Ann.av. 24-h ($\mu g/m^3$)	40.5 (4.7)
Ozone (8-hours $\mu g/m^3$)	Ann.av. 8-hour ($\mu g/m^3$)	62.7 (32.0)
Environmental Tobacco Smoke	Prevalence	
Nonsmoking men 1970	Smoking partner	0.26
Nonsmoking women 1970	Smoking partner	0.60
Nonsmoking men 1990	Smoking partner	0.22
Nonsmoking women 1990	Smoking partner	0.30
Children 1995	Smoking house	0.40
Damp homes	Prevalence	0.175 (0.07)

Dutch ministry of housing (de Hollander and Staatsen, 2003). Based on an extensive monitoring programme in more than 1,500 Dutch dwellings, (future) exposure to indoor radon of the Dutch population was modelled based on characteristics of the total stock of dwellings, such as air-tightness, building materials and ventilation behaviour (de Hollander and Staatsen, 2003; National Institute of Public Health and the Environment, 2000).

6.2. *Long-term Versus Short-term Mortality*

For the sake of clarity (and simplicity), we make a distinction between exogenous risk factors that are involved in the onset and progression of (chronic) disease and risk factors that primarily "accelerate" death among the weak. The first type of interaction can be shown in cohort studies, in which populations are followed up during a sufficiently long period to see whether certain exposures affect the incidence or mortality of disease, allowing for gender, age, smoking, occupational status and diet. Examples of these are studies among workers exposed to hazardous substances in an occupational setting (i.e. radon, benzene and polycyclic aromatic hydrocarbons) and a number of American cohort studies retrospectively relating survival among citizens to air pollution levels (Dockery *et al.*, 1993; Pope III *et al.*, 1995; Abbey *et al.*, 1999; Lipfert *et al.*, 2003). Results of both the American Cancer Society Cohort (ACS) and the Harvard Six Cities studies stood up to extensive scrutiny by the Health Effects Institute (Krewski *et al.*, 2000). An extension of the follow-up of the ACS study yielded results that were consistent with earlier reports (Pope III *et al.*, 2002). Therefore, it is reasonable to assume that long-term exposure to particulate air pollution indeed affects survival, especially by increasing the risk of cardiopulmonary disease and lung cancer. "Harvesting", the bringing forward of death among the susceptible, for instance, through aggravation of disease during unfavourable air pollution conditions, would go unnoticed in this type of study, given the extended "time-window" of many years. This effect is especially seen in time series analysis, observing day-to-day variations (Brunekreef, 1997; Künzli *et al.*, 2001). Nonetheless, the accumulation of these day-to-day health insults underlying changes in mortality and hospital admission alone may very well be the cause of chronic morbidity and survival loss (World Health Organization, 2003).

To estimate loss of life-years, we applied the concept of attributable risk, assuming that cause-specific mortality due to environmental exposure is similar to any "other" cause-specific mortality, with respect to onset and time of dying. For each end-point, we estimated the years of life lost by means of life-table analysis (i.e. the sum of number of cases per age-group times remaining life expectancy divided by total number of cases), similar to previous work on *national* average life-expectancy (Brunekreef, 1997; Nevalainen and Pekkanen, 1998; Leksell and Rabl, 2001). We also investigated the sensitivity of the result to changing relative risks with age or implementing a certain length follow-up (Table 6).

Several sophisticated epidemiological analyses have been undertaken to estimate the loss of life-years due to the short-term mortality that is revealed by the analysis of time series of daily mortality and air pollution data. Most analyses suggest the average loss of lifetime would range from a few days to several months. In some cases, the loss may extend to one year or more, for instance, due to pneumonia or heart attacks (Schwartz, 1998; Zeger *et al.*, 1999; Zanobetti *et al.*, 2002; Dominici *et al.*, 2003). Furthermore, several analyses have shown that most of the air pollution associated deaths occur outside the hospital, implying that these effects are not limited to the terminally ill (Schwartz, 1994). We will apply a rather non-informative subjective distribution here, ranging from one day to ten years, with an average of three months (Table 6).

As in the case of long-term mortality, here we apply the concept of population attributable risk. The fraction attributable to air pollution exposure is assumed to be similar to the total morbidity load. To assess the time spent with a certain morbidity, we use annual prevalence data (asthma, ischaemic heart disease). In a stable situation by definition, prevalence equals the number of new cases times the average duration of the condition (Melse and Kramers, 1999).

Estimates for the duration of health care events were either derived from the literature, the Dutch health care registration (NIVEL) or from expert consultation (van Schayck *et al.*, 199?; Barnes *et al.*, 1996; Taylor and Newacheck, 1992; Burney, 1996; Krahn *et al.*, 1996). An overview of duration estimates is presented in Table 6.

6.3. *The Health Market*

To assess the loss of economic utility associated with the health endpoints involved, one would require an economic valuation of the full quality of life impact to the affected individual. This would include expenses such as medical costs and lost income (often referred to

Table 6.   Estimated duration of effects of particles.

Health Response (Particulate Matter, PM_{10})	Distribution Applied in Monte Carlo Analysis	Parameters (years)
Long term mortality	**(Dutch life table)**	
Overall annual mortality	no	10.9
Cardiopulmonary	no	8.2
Lung cancer	no	13.0
Ischaemic heart disease	**subjective Beta[a]**	
	minimum	0.0027
	most likely	0.5
	mean	1
	maximum	11.3
Sudden infant death	no	70
Daily mortality	**subjective Beta[b]**	
	minimum	0.0027
	most likely	0.083
	mean	0.25
	maximum	10
Hospital admission	**subjective Beta[c]**	
Respiratory	minimum	0.011
Cardio-vascular	most likely	0.019
	mean	0.038
	maximum	0.167
Emergency room visits	**normal**	
Respiratory	mean	0.033
	stand. dev.	0.021
Aggravation of asthma	**uniform**	
Attacks	min	0.0027
Use of bronchodilators	max	0.0055
Respiratory symptoms	**point estimate**	
Upper respiratory tract		0.019
Lower respiratory tract		0.038
Lung cancer morbidity	**point estimate[d]**	2.9

[a]A subjective Beta distribution incorporating the following quantitative assumptions: Minimum loss of life expectancy 1 day, most likely half a year, average 1 year, maximum 11.3, the latter being the loss based on life-table calculation (passive smoking as dominant cause of morbidity and death).
[b]A subjective Beta distribution incorporating the following quantitative assumptions: Minimum loss of life expectancy 1 day, most likely a month, average 3 months, maximum 10 years, being the loss based on life-table calculation (the unlikely possibility air pollution is the dominant cause of morbidity and death).
[c]A subjective Beta distribution incorporating the following expert assumptions: Minimum duration of disease aggravation episode 4 days, most likely one week, average two weeks, maximum two months.
[d]Based on Dutch data on incidence and prevalence (Ruwaard and Kramers, 1998).

as cost of illness, COI), and less tangible effects on well-being such as pain, discomfort and restriction of everyday activities. One way of assessing the economic utility loss is to ascertain the individual maximum WTP for the reduced incidence of illness and adverse symptoms. To compile a set of WTP-values for the health impacts quantified, we drew upon a number of studies that reviewed the literature on WTP for avoiding changes in the risk of death, chronic diseases as well as milder morbidity effects (Krupnick and Portney, 1991; Ostro and Chestnut, 1998; Aunan *et al.*, 1998; Holland *et al.*, 1998; USEPA, 1996; Institute for Environmental Studies, 1997). These values were primarily derived from studies in which preferences of both healthy and infirm individuals were revealed through questionnaires, the "so-called" contingent valuation studies. In some cases, in the absence of reliable data, COI estimates were used as a proxy, adjusted upwards by a factor of 2. Table 7 lists the WTP values derived from these reviews. From a review of these studies, we suggest a range for the value of a (statistical) death of EUR 2–7 million, with a central estimate of around EUR 4,500,000. The contingency valuation method produces the highest estimates, while the consumer market studies yield the lowest values (Holland *et al.*, 1998).

The economic valuation of daily mortality presents a problem as most reviews suggest that recorded deaths may often involve old people suffering from severe chronic disease ("harvesting"). Compared with fatalities among young or middle aged healthy individuals, a number of adjustments are justified concerning loss of life-years, average age distribution, and the quality of life of the cases involved. Much in accordance with the report of the Ad-Hoc Group on the Economic Appraisal of the Health Effects of Air Pollution in the UK (Ad-Hoc group, 1999), we propose a lower limit of EUR 1,200 using a maximum reduction factor adjusting for loss of life-years, age and disability (i.e. 0.083: assuming a minimum individual loss of life expectancy of one week instead of 12 year; 0.75 to adjust for a lower valuation of a prevented statistical fatality at older ages (Holland *et al.*, 1998; Jones-Lee, 1985), and 0.2 as the lower bound of the disability weight for the very ill) (Ad-Hoc group, 1999). The upper bound estimate of the value of a prevented statistical fatality would equal the unadjusted (central) estimate, given the unlikely possibility that daily mortality

Table 7. Monetary values for health endpoints based on "willingness to pay" (WTP).

Health Response (Particulate Matter, PM_{10})	Distribution	Euros
Long term mortality	**discrete**	
Overall annual mortality	lower (0.33)	1,950,000
Cardiopulmonary	middle (0.5)	4,360,000
Lung cancer	upper (0.17)	6,760,000
Ischaemic heart disease		
Sudden infant death		
Chronic bronchitis	**discrete**	
	lower (0.33)	150,000[a]
	middle (0.33)	220,000
	upper (0.33)	390,000
Asthma	**discrete**	
	lower (0.33)	65,000[b]
	middle (0.33)	105,000
	upper (0.33)	130,000
Chronic respir sympt (1 year)	**discrete**	
	lower (0.33)	165[c]
	middle (0.33)	330
	upper (0.33)	495
Daily mortality	**subjective Beta**	
	minimum	1,200[d]
	most likely	36,000
	mean	109,000
	maximum	4,360,000
Hospital admission	**discrete**	
Respiratory	lower (0.33)	1,100[e]
	middle (0.33)	7,000
	upper (0.33)	14,000
Cardio-vascular	lower (0.33)	1,100[e]
	middle (0.33)	7,000
	upper (0.33)	15,000
Emergency room visits	**discrete**	
Respiratory	lower (0.33)	260[f]
	middle (0.33)	520
	upper (0.33)	780

(*Continued*)

Table 7. (*Continued*)

Health Response (Particulate Matter, PM_{10})	Distribution	Euros
Aggravation of asthma	**discrete**	
Attacks	lower (0.33)	35[g]
Use of bronchodilators	middle (0.33)	70
	upper (0.33)	140
Respiratory symptoms	**discrete**	
Upper respiratory tract	lower (0.33)	6[h]
	middle (0.33)	12
	upper (0.33)	18
Lower respiratory tract	**discrete**	
	lower (0.33)	6[i]
	middle (0.33)	38
	upper (0.33)	330

[a]Based on contingent valuation study in the US (Ostro and Chestnut, 1998; Viscusi *et al.*, 1991).

[b]Based on contingent valuation study in the US (Ostro and Chestnut, 1998; Holland *et al.*, 1998).

[c]Based on adjusted Cost of illness (COI) for cases of acute bronchitis in the US (Ostro and Chestnut, 1998).

[d]See text (Ad-Hoc group, 1999).

[e]Lower estimate based on empirical relationship between WTP and quality of life in accordance with Ref. 21; central estimate based on contingent valuation study in the US (Holland, *et al.*, 1998); upper estimate adjusted COI in the US (Ostro and Chestnut, 1998).

[f]Based on WTP-study in the US (Ostro and Chestnut, 1998; Holland *et al.*, 1998).

[g]Lower estimate WTP from adjusted COI (Ostro and Chestnut, 1998); central estimate WTP non-asthmatic respondents, upper estimate WTP asthmatic respondents in Norwegian CVM-study (Navrud, 1997).

[h]Based on CVM-estimates in the US (Ostro and Chestnut, 1998) and a Norwegian study (Navrud, 1997).

[i]Lower estimate based on CVM-study in the US (Ostro and Chestnut, 1998); central estimate based on Norwegian study (Navrud, 1997); upper estimate WTP for acute bronchitis in the US (Ostro and Chestnut, 1998).

would involve a healthy subject with an average life expectancy. For the "mean" and "most likely" monetary estimates, the loss of life-time per case is assumed to be 6 and 2 months respectively; a factor of 0.6 is applied to adjust for age and disability (Davis *et al.*, 2002).

As immediate benefits are in general more valuable to people than future benefits, many valuation systems used in cost-benefit analysis apply discount rates not just for costs, but for health benefits as well (e.g. 3% annually). As we did not make a formal cost-effectiveness analysis, we have not applied discount rates in this instance. In our exercise, discount rates would apply to chronic effects such as premature mortality or an extra case of chronic bronchitis. A discount rate of 3% over 10 years would reduce the valuation in DALYs or Euros by around 13%. This would fall well within the range of uncertainty we deal with in this analysis.

6.4. *Uncertainty*

We analysed the uncertainty in the calculations of air pollution related DALYs and Euros by means of Monte Carlo techniques (Burmaster and Anderson, 1994; Hoffman and Hammonds, 1994; Thompson *et al.*, 1992). In a Monte Carlo simulation model, input parameters are treated as random variables. For each of the input parameters such as population exposure, exposure-response function estimates, average duration of the response and discount factors, a probability distributions function was estimated, representing parameter uncertainty. Subsequently, an output distribution for the different health impact measures was estimated by iterative (Latin hypercube) sampling from each of the defined parameter distributions, followed by recalculation. We will present the 5th and 95th percentiles of this distribution as a measure of uncertainty in this case.

7. Deaths, DALYs and Dollars (Euro)

Point estimates as well as the 5th and 95th percentiles of the probability distribution for impact metrics are shown as a measure of uncertainty (Table 8, Fig. 4). In most cases, this uncertainty range is substantial but less than one order of magnitude (Burmaster and Anderson, 1994; Hoffman and Hammonds, 1994; Thompson *et al.*, 1992).

Table 8. Summary of health impact estimates for a number of air pollution phenomenon, expressed in fatalities, DALYs and Euros.

Environmental Factor	Health Outcome	#/million[a]	5-95%-tile	DALYs million	5-95%-tile	Euros (x10^6)/million	5-95%-tile
Particulate Air pollution Long-term	*Mortality*						
	- Cardiopulmonary	135	61-221	781	252-1,462	585	235-1,056
	- Lung cancer	30	-58-113	270	-525-1,136	130	-256-520
	Morbidity						
	- Chronic resp. sympt.	3,660	961-6,780	147	33-303	1.2	0.3-2.4
	- Chronic bronchitis	458	109-805	1,201	265-2,307	116	25-222
Total long term		215[b]	71-384	2,020	1,080-3,931	834	282-1,440
Particulate Air pollution Short-term	*Mortality*						
	- Respiratory	12	7-17	2	0.2-5.8	1.3	0.1-3.4
	- Coronary heart dis.	25	11-41	4.4	0.4-12.6	2.8	0.3-7.7
	- Pneumonia	7.8	4.5-11.5	1.4	0.1-3.8	0.9	0.1-2.3
	- Other	41.3	7.5-77.5	7.2	0.4-22.4	4.5	0.2-13.8
	Hospital admission						
	- Respiratory	100	50-170	2.2	0.8-4.3	0.7	0.2-1.5
	- Cardiovascular	101	49-175	2.5	0.9-4.8	0.8	0.2-1.6
	Emergency room visits						
	- Respiratory	1,800	610-3,400	29	4-75	0.9	0.3-1.9
	Aggravation of asthma						
	- Asthmatic attacks	5,6000	7,500-125,000	31	2-86	4.6	0.6-11
	- Use of bronchodil.	60,000	7,600-136,000	33	2.1-93	5	0.6-12
	Aggravation of resp. symptoms						
	- Upper resp tract	11,500	1,500-22,600	9.7	0-28	0.1	0-0.3
	- Lower resp tract	4,600	1,040-8,500	30	2.5-85	0.6	0.1-1.5
	Affected lung function						
Total short term		87[b]	16-162	120	54-208	17	9-29
Ozone	*Mortality*						
	- Respiratory	21	4-50	3.8	0.2-12.8	2.4	0.2-7.6
	- Cardiovascular	47	5-140	8.1	0.3-29	5.1	0.2-19
	- Pneumonia	11	1-26	1.9	0-6.7	1.2	0-4.1
	- Other	75	0-250	13	0-61	8.2	0-36

(*Continued*)

Table 8.   (*Continued*)

Environmental Factor	Health Outcome	#/million[a]	5–95%-tile	DALYs million	5–95%-tile	Euros (x106)/million	5–95%-tile
	Hospital admission						
	- Respiratory disease	86	−10–207	2.5	−0.3–6.3	0.6	−0.1–1.7
	Emergency room visits						
	- Respiratory disease	1,540	−150–4,200	25	−2.1–83	0.8	−0.1–2.3
Total ozone		154	32–328	54	9.5–131	18.2	2.5–48
Damp houses	*Asthma*						
	- Children	1,665	898–2,622	133	58–235	41	21–68
	- Adults	1,814	683–3,430	145	47–302	45	16–87
	Lower resp disease						
	- Children	661	300–1,165	27	5.6–61	0.5	0.2–1.1
	- Adults	6,092	3,140–9,730	250	53–520	5	1.9–9.2
Total dampness		0	0	554	300–880	92	53–142
ETS	lung cancer–morbid.	1.9	1.3–2.4	0.8	0.5–1.2		
	(female)–mortality	0.9	0.6–1.2	12.2	8.5–15.7	2.8	1.9–3.7
	lung cancer–morbid.	2.7	0.7–4.7	1.2	5–45		
	(male)–mortality	1.3	0.3–2.3	17	4.5–30.5	3.9	1.0–7.1
	IHD						
	- Morbidity females	118	75–162	34	17–55		
	- Mortality females	16.5	10.4–23	90	22–175	50	32–71
	- Morbidity males	116	73–162	34	17–54		
	- Mortality males	15	9.5–21	83	21–161	47	29–66
	- Aggravation of asthma	91,780	42,720–1,538,200	51	9–118	3.4	1.3–6.3
	Lower resp symptoms	1,900	1,600–2,150	12	1.5–28	0.2	0.0–0.5
	- Otitis media acuta	2,700	1,250–4,100	30	1.1–76	0.3	0.1–0.8
	Sudden infant death	0.6	0.1–1.1	43	5–76	1.9	0.2–3.4
Total ETS		35	26–43	410	280–553	110	84–139
Radon	Lung cancer morbid	22	13–32	95	56–134	33	19–47
	Lung cancer mort	10.6	6.2–15	9.6	5.2–14.8		
Total radon		35	26–43	105	62–148	33	19–47
Overall		261	85–458	3,220	1,825–4,780	990	440–1,600

[a]Number of people affected.
[b]Number of death only.

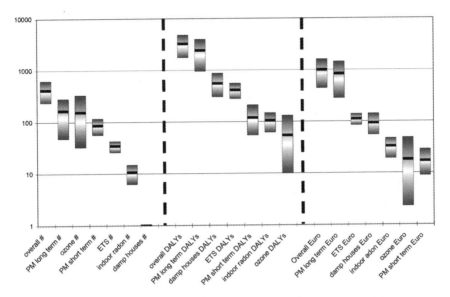

Fig. 4. Annual health loss for a number of air pollution phenomenon expressed in terms of fatality numbers (left hand panel), DALYs (central panel) and millionEuros per million inhabitants (right hand panel). Box plots show point estimates and 5th and 95th percentile values.

In our calculations, the health loss related to air pollution is substantially dominated by the long-term effects of particulate air pollution, which amounts to 37% of deaths, 67% of total DALY-loss and 76% of the total monetary loss related to air pollution (Table 8). The estimated "monetarised" loss is huge, almost EUR 16 billion (5–95%-tiles: 7–25 billion), which is between one quarter and one third of the total annual budget for Health Care in the Netherlands, but it must be stressed that this is only an indicative figure, as the WTP-amount of money is not "real money".

Over the past decade, annual investments in traffic emission reduction in the Netherlands totalled between EUR 250 and 350 million, yielding an emission reduction of around 4% per year (Central Bareau of Statistics, 2003). If we assume that there is a linear relation between emission and actual population exposure, the benefits of these investments in terms of monetarised health gain are in the same order of magnitude, if not higher (i.e. 4% of an annual disease burden of EUR 13 billion: EUR 550 million). Based on the same assumption, the cost of air pollution control measures per DALY saved is around EUR 100,000. In recent discussions among health economists, an investment of EUR 40,000 to 50,000 for each equivalent year of perfect health gained by an intervention is regarded as "acceptable value for money" (Towse *et al.*, 2002). The World Bank recently proposed 3 times the Gross Domestic Product per capita; for the Netherlands, that would be approximately EUR 75,000/DALY saved.

The total air pollution attributable disease burden is estimated to be in the order of 50,000 (5–95%-tiles: 25,000–75,000) DALYs annually. As expected, the health loss attributable to environmental exposures is relatively small in the Netherlands. Recently, the total annual burden of disease was estimated to be in the order of 2.6 million DALYs (Ruwaard and Kramers, 1998). According to the calculations presented here, the air pollution impact described here would contribute slightly less than 2% of the total disease burden. In the Netherlands, life-style factors such as smoking, unfavourable eating habits and physical inactivity cause a much greater burden of disease, i.e. 14.7, 8.5 and 6.6 of total disease burden (DALYs) respectively (de Hollander, 2003).

The metric used to express air pollution associated health loss, mortality risk, DALYs or Euros has an obvious effect on the rank order of the different types of air pollution effect (Fig. 5). The high mortality counts associated with air pollution episodes are not reflected in the amounts of lost DALYs and Euro, as a substantial part of it is considered to be due to "harvesting" of those with only a limited time to live. No mortality is calculated for damp houses, but chronic bronchitis associated with damp housing weighs heavily in terms of DALYs and Euro.

In Fig. 6, for each air pollution exposure, the disease burden in DALYs is plotted against monetarised health loss on a log-scale. On average the DALY is worth around EUR 300,000, but the plot is clearly very scattered.

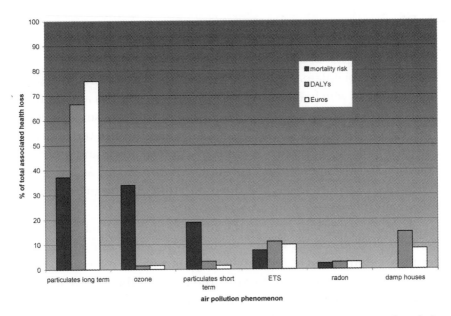

Fig. 5. Overview of health impact of air pollution type as percentages of total air health loss expressed in terms of fatality numbers, DALYs and Euro.

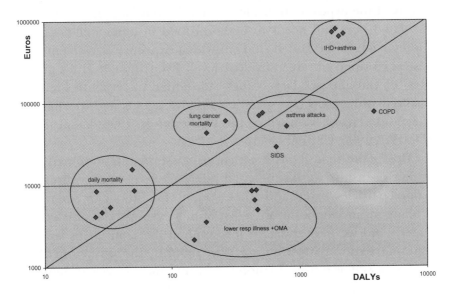

Fig. 6. Response specific DALYs plotted against response specific Euros.

8. Discussion

8.1. *Health Impact Assessment*

Several potential flaws are associated with this type of impact assessment, most of which are not specific to the approaches and metrics we have proposed here, but concern health impact assessment in general. Recurring, almost inevitable shortcomings involve the imprecision of population exposure assessments, the unknown, and probably "unknowable" shape of the exposure-response curves at low, environmental exposure levels, and the translation of exposure-response information from one population to another.

Another important issue is the internal and external validity of epidemiological results. In view of the way in which our aggregated results are dominated by the long-term public health effects of particulate air pollution, we have to stress the fact that these estimates are only based on the results of two American cohort studies and a small Dutch pilot study (Dockery *et al.*, 1993; Pope III *et al.*, 1995; Abbey *et al.*; Hoek *et al.*, 2002). Given the inherent shortcomings of this type of retrospective epidemiological study, especially with respect to the validity of the exposure indicators, the relatively large health impact calculated here still needs to be confirmed in other well-designed studies, such as the Dutch study in which exposure assessment is at least performed on an individual level. Even though Hill's guidelines for causality are largely met, substantial uncertainties remain unsolved with respect to specific causative agents and mechanism of actions (Health Council of the Netherlands, 1996; Vedal, 1997; COMEAP, 1995; USEPA, 1996).

Most of the quantitative health impact assessments presented here are fairly sensitive to the choice of reference level of exposure. Suspended particles, ozone and other oxidants in outdoor air and radon or allergens in indoor air are a fact of life, even without any human activity; and we have more or less applied the concept of feasible minimum exposure distribution. If we optimise the way we build our houses as well as our ventilation behaviour, radon levels should not exceed 16 Bq/m^3 and damp houses would be very rare. In principle, a world without smokers is possible (be it not imaginable), so exposure may be zero. For particulates (PM$_{10}$) and ozone, we tentatively applied 15 and 20 μg/m^3 as the baseline exposure levels.

The most fundamental problem we encountered was a lack of complete and quantitative insights into how air pollutant exposures are involved in the onset and development of human disease. We have only incorporated exposure-response associations, which have been studied comprehensively in epidemiological research and for which clearly defined health outcomes have been established. "Health events" that are recorded in epidemiological surveys or health care registration may only be the tip of the iceberg, with many minor impairments remaining undetected beneath the surface (see Fig. 1) (de Hollander and Staatsen, 2003). In particular, time-series analyses provide us with the means to detect relatively small elevations of mortality and hospital admission during episodes. It is almost inconceivable that these relatively severe health events would occur without susceptibility in the population suffering from transient lung function deficits, or asthma or angina attacks, resulting in an increased use of medication, or visits to the general practitioner or the emergency room. However, obvious means of investigation, such as panel studies appear to lack sufficient power to detect an increased incidence of such endpoints (Brunekreef and Holgate, 2002; Roemer *et al.*, 2000).

8.2. *Environmental Health Impacts on a Scale*

Attributing impact weights to air pollution related conditions involve societal and individual values and preferences, which do not always agree well with the scientific traditions in several disciplines. At the same time, normative evaluation of health-endpoints is virtually inevitable in health risk assessment. Even using annual mortality risk as an impact measure is value-laden, as non-fatal health outcomes as well as age at death (loss of life expectancy) are implicitly ignored. The same applies for health-based exposure guidelines, for which value judgements have to be made regarding the health significance of toxicological or epidemiological response variables.

Whose values matter and how are these best assessed? A large number of studies have revealed that the health-related quality weights attributed to certain health states may differ between patients and non-patients (de Wit *et al.*, 2000). Health status weights for DALYs are mostly derived by calling in health professionals, who are able to assess the various dimensions of disease. WTP-values are determined with the help of large-scale surveys. Both have their own systematic biases, but policy decisions about resource allocation should adopt a societal perspective and may thus involve these types of generic preference classifications. Furthermore, it is important to notice that health preference measurements tend to be rather stable and reproducible, even across countries (Melse and de Hollander, 2001; Department of Health, 1998).

In health economics, there are five main ways to elucidate preferences with respect to health status quality, i.e. standard gamble (choosing between probabilities of possible outcome), time trade-off (exchanging time with different health states), person trade-off (exchanging persons with different health states), contingent valuation and revealed preference (wage-risk, hedonic pricing etc.). Results produced by different methods may differ substantially indicating that many socio-psychological processes are not accounted for. An appealing example is that most people find it impossible to exchange relatively minor morbidity outcomes among many with death among a few (e.g. reluctance to give up life). Several authors have claimed that real-life preferences with respect to health and life expectancy are much too complicated to be covered by the simple concept of DALY. They argue that the plain observation that preferences are not stable over a life-time and will depend largely on whether health states will occur near or far into the future, makes application of DALYs questionable. Others favour the more pragmatic approach that there are simply no better alternatives (Hurley, 2000).

Uncertainty analysis shows that altering weights within the variance seen in most weighting exercises does not substantially affect the overall picture. Compared with the huge uncertainties that are often connected with health impact estimates, the effect of the possible variance in attributed weights appears rather small. However, there is an important exception. The lower the disability weights attributed to health states, the more sensitive they are to variation. It is much easier to double the small weight given to severe noise annoyance than to double that of the terminal state of lung cancer. This is reflected in the results of the uncertainty analysis with respect to "respiratory illness". The variation of the output probability distribution is largely due to variation in the severity weights given by panel members. Since the less severe responses tend to affect the highest number of people, there is some room for "manipulation" of results, e.g. increasing the public health significance of "one's favourite health risk".

8.3. *Worth the Money?*

The calculations with respect to the monetary valuation of air pollution health impacts indicate an enormous loss in economic terms. However, the loss is primarily due to the long-term effects on survival associated with particle exposure, of which the validity is still debated. This dilemma of uncertain health impacts yielding a huge health loss stresses the necessity to complete the economic appraisal with accepted methods for economic valuation of uncertainty (Holland *et al.*, 1998; Ad-Hoc group, 1999).

As already mentioned, the transfer of WTP-values from other studies can be tricky, since valuations may be largely determined by contextual variables, comprising risk perception or the respondent's perspective (i.e. individual versus collective, altruistic versus self-centred). An economic appraisal of air pollution health effects may profit from WTP-estimates based on European contingent valuation studies that directly concern air pollution health effects in the right context.

Air pollution attributable health loss expressed in DALYs is not completely proportional to the health loss in terms of Euros (Fig. 6), although there is some convergence. Theoretically, this might be explained by the fact that both measures are based on different principles. Monetary valuation may involve all possible dimensions of reduced health, while DALYs are an aggregate of only three formal dimensions, number of people involved, duration and severity. Health responses to exposures that are dominated by mortality, such as the impacts of ozone and particles (long-term) produce relatively higher health loss estimates for Euros than for DALYs, and vice versa for short-term responses and morbidity due to particles. Of course, one has to bear in mind that many shortcomings are connected to an economic appraisal of the prevention of statistical fatalities as well as morbidity risks. For instance, the wage-risk method relies on the assumption of enough labour mobility for workers to really have a free choice, which is doubtful in most cases (Holland *et al.*, 1998). With respect to the contingent valuation method producing general WTP figures, a number of objections have been raised. In the first place, it is a highly hypothetical number, i.e. it is not real money but simply what people claim they would spend in this "virtual" market place. Secondly, respondents may also show "strategic" behaviour. People with "green" preferences may intentionally exaggerate their willingness to pay; others may provide interviewers with politically correct answers. Thirdly, respondents may feel it is unethical to put a price tag on someone else's death or illness, and lastly, given the often-complex nature of the questionnaires, contingent valuation methods are vulnerable to many potential biases ("starting point bias", "interviewer bias", and "embedding bias"). Some health end-points may be rather hypothetical to most of the respondents, but at the same time familiar to others, e.g. asthmatic attacks. Familiarity with end-points such as asthmatic attacks and chronic bronchitis appears to increase WTP (Davis *et al.*, 2002; Kruppnick and Cropper, 1992).

Thus, there is reason for concern about the stability of the quantitative preferences of respondents, for which we have only limited insight into. For instance, many risk perception studies underline the importance of context variables such as personal interest in risk source, perceived personal and institutional control over risk generating activities, degree of voluntariness of exposure and inequity with respect to distribution of risks and benefits (Slovic, 1999). Other socio-economic and demographic variables may also be important, such as base-line risk or personal income and education. This type of uncertainty may not fully justify the transfer of WTP-measurements to health impact assessment of air pollution. In particular, most of the WTP-studies involving morbidity risks have been done in the US and there are systematic differences between the US and Europe in the cultural and socio-economic dimensions discussed here. Consequently, the results of WTP-calculations should be regarded as crude estimates, allowing comparisons between different risks rather than regarding the costs as real money.

In the framework of this study, we have not fully considered the feasibility or costs of measures to reduce air pollutant exposure. It is clear that current ambient air concentration of particles and ozone can only be reduced at high economic and societal costs, while a certain level must be considered as a fact of life. For environmental tobacco smoke and dampness in homes, measures to reduce population exposure may be less expensive for a comparable benefit, although data on these indoor factors are lacking in this context.

8.4. *Equity and Efficiency*

It is important to note here that the choice of an indicator to represent environmental health loss is not just an academic question. It is not just coincidence or lack of methodology that lies in the choice of mortality risk as the classical health loss indicator. Managing risk based on mortality guarantees that everybody is equally treated, but simple application of health adjusted life-years as a measure of health impact is not without serious distribution or ethical consequences. In principle, society would benefit from passing health risks to the elderly, since they have less life-years and health to lose. Furthermore, the use of DALYs implies that people with a disease count is less than that of the healthy people. In this respect, some authors warn against double jeopardy, where people with poor health suffer a disadvantage twice. Firstly, they are disabled and secondly, the saving of one year of their lives counts less than that of an healthy person. One can strive to maximise utility, but one can also strive to concentrate efforts on people with the worst health, or those with the greatest improvement potential (Nord, 1999).

WTP-values are also dependent on income. Application of WTP may thus violate equity principles, especially when locally-derived WTP values are applied globally, typically giving less weight to third world health problems (Hofstetter and Hammitt, 2002).

8.5. *Conclusion*

In spite of methodological and ethical problems, presenting health impact in terms of DALYs and/or money offers a promising framework for *explicit evaluation* and *comparison* of health loss associated with different environmental exposures, involving a wide variety of non-fatal health outcomes. It enables incorporation of the public health interest in decision making with respect to environmental quality and spatial planning (e.g. extensive infrastructure projects involving a range of diverging, often accumulating exposures). For instance, in scenario studies, aggregates can be applied to explore the "health" score of different options, evaluated from the perspective of different policy philosophies.

The calculation of DALYs associated with environmental exposures provides a comparative picture from the viewpoint of public health. However, we would not suggest an immediate change of environmental policy priorities based on this type of calculation. Policy priorities may be partly explained by dimensions of health risk perception which are not captured in our approach, such as "dread", voluntariness of exposure, the perceived controllability or familiarity of risk generating processes (e.g. traffic). In particular, the social distribution of risk and benefit (Slovic, 1999) is not covered in our approach, as by definition, a slight reduction of health amongst many may be equal to severely affected health amongst a few. From the viewpoint of policy makers, the principle of equity may prevail.

Application of monetary valuation of health-endpoints in principle allows formal cost-benefit analysis of policy options to improve the air pollution situation from different perspectives. As further air pollution control becomes increasingly expensive, affecting individual behaviour rather than institutions (e.g. the energy or industrial sector), a crude indication of what we are willing to pay to avoid health impacts attributable to air pollution may improve the policy making process. However, this would necessitate more adequate WTP-estimates, preferably from European studies explicitly dealing with air pollution situations.

Application of aggregate health metrics, such as DALYs and WTP, can be of help in environmental health policy as long as they are not considered as the ultimate "health coin", and as long as other criteria, such as equity and solidarity, are incorporated in decision making as well.

Acknowledgement

We thank Bert Brunekreef, Bernard van de Berg and Eltjo Buringh for their critical comments on the manuscript.

References

Abbey D.E., Nishino N., McDonnell W.F., Burchette R.J., Knutsen S.F., Beeson W.I. and Yang J.X. Long-term inhalable particles and other air pollutants related to mortality in non-smokers.

Abbey D.E., Nishino N., McDonnell W.F., Burchette R.J., Knutsen S.F., Lawrence-Beeson W. and Yang J.X. (1999) Long-term inhalable particles and other air pollutants related to mortality in nonsmokers. *Am J Respir Crit Care Med* **159**(2): 373–382.

Abbey D.E., Ostro B.E., Petersen F. and Burchette R.J. (1995) Chronic respiratory symptoms associated with estimated long-term ambient concentrations of fine particulates less than 2.5 microns in aerodynamic diameter (PM2.5) and other air pollutants. *J Expo Anal Environ Epidemiol* **5**(2): 137–159.

Abbey D.E., Petersen F., Mills P.K. and Beeson W.L. (1993) Long-term ambient concentrations of total suspended particulates, ozone and sulfur dioxine and respiratory symptoms in a non-smoking population. *Arch Environ Health* **18**(1): 33–46.

Ad-Hoc group on the economic appraisal of the health effects of air pollution. Economic appraisal of the health effects of air pollution. HMSO, London, 1999.

Aunan K. (1996) Exposure-response functions for health efects of air pollutants based on epidemiological findings. *Risk Anal* **16**: 693–709.

Aunan K., Pátzay G., Asbjørn Aaheim H. and Martin Seip H. (1998) Health and environmental benefits from air pollution reductions in Hungary. *Sci Total Environ* **212**: 245–268.

Barnes P.J. and Jonsson Klim J.B. (1996) The costs of asthma. *Eur Respir J* **9**: 636–642.

Bell M.L. and Davis D.L. Reassessment of the lethal London fog of 1952: Novel indicators of acute and chronic consequences of acute exposure to air pollution. *Environ Health Perspect* 2001; **109**(suppl 3): 389–394.

Brunekreef B. (1997) Air pollution and life expectancy: Is there a relation? *Occup Environ Med* **54**: 781–784.

Brunekreef B. (1999) All but quiet on the particulate front (editorial). *Am J Respir Crit Care Med* **158**: 354–356.

Brunekreef B. and Holgate S.T. (2002) Air pollution and health. Review. *Lancet* **360**: 1233–1242.

Burmaster D.E. and Anderson P.D. (1994) Principles of good practice for the use of Monte Carlo techniques in human health and ecological risk assessment. *Risk Anal* **14**: 477–481.

Burney P. (eds). (1996) Variations in the prevalence of respiratory symptoms, self-reported asthma attacks, and use of asthma medication in the European Community Respiratory Health Survey (ECRHS). *Eur Respir J* **9**: 687–695.

Central Bureau of Statistics. Voorburg/Heerlen, 2003: http://statline.cbs.nl.

COMEAP. Non-biological particles and Health. HSMO Committee on the Medical Effects of Air Pollution, London. 1995.

Davis D.L., Krupnick A. and Thurston G. The ancillary health benefits and costs of CHG mitigation: Scope, scale and credibility. Resources for the Future, 2002 (www.rff.org).

de Mills P.K., Petersen F.F. and Beeson W.L. (1991) Long-term ambient concentrations of total suspended particulates and oxidants as related to incidence of chronic disease in California Seventh-Day Adventists. *Environ Health Perspect* **94**: 43–50.

Department of Health: Committee on the Medical Effects of Air Pollutants (COMEAP). Quantification of the effects of air pollution on health in the United Kingdom. HMSO, London.

Diener A., O'Brien B. and Gafni A. (1998) Health care contingent valuation studies: A review and classification of the literature. *Health Econ* **7**(4): 313–326.

Dockery D.W. and Pope III C.A. (1994) Acute respiratory effects of particulate air pollution. *Annu Rev Public Health* **15**: 107–132.

Dockery D.W., Pope III C.A., Xu X., Spengler J.D., Ware J.H., Fay M.E., *et al.* (1993) An association between air pollution and mortality in six US cities. *N Engl J Med* **340**: 1010–1014.

Dockery D.W., Speizer F.E., Stram D.O., Ware J.H., Spengler J.D. and Ferris B.G. (1989) Effects of inhalable particles on respiratory health in children. *Am Rev Respir Dis* **139**: 587–594.

Dominici F., McDermott A., Zeger S.L. and Samet J.M. (2003) Airborne particulate matter and mortality: Timescale effects in four US cities. *Am J Epidemiol* **157**: 1055–1065.

Dutch Foundation on Smoking and Health (StiVoRo). Annual Report (in Dutch). Den Haag: StiVoRo, 1998.

Eerens H.C., Sliggers C.J., van den Hout K.D. (1993) The CAR model: The Dutch method to determine city street air quality. *Atmos Environ* **27B**: 389–399.

Essink-Bot M.L. Health status as a measure of outcome of disease treatment. Erasmus University Rotterdam (Thesis), 1995.

Gerdtham U.G. and Johannesson M. (2002) Do life-saving regulations safe lives? *J Risk Uncertainty* **24**: 231–249.

Hammitt J.K. (2002) QALYs versus WTP. *Risk Anal* **22**: 985–1001.

Health Council of the Netherlands: Committee on Risk Measures and Risk Assessment. Risk is more than just a number. The Hague: Health Council of the Netherlands, 1996; publication no. 1996/03E.

Health Council of the Netherlands: Committee on Risk Measures and Risk Assessment. Risk is more than just a number. The Hague: Health Council of the Netherlands, 1996; publication no. 1996/03E.

Hoek G. and Brunekreef B. (1993) Acute effects of a winter air pollution episode on pulmonary function and respiratory symptoms of children. *Arch-Environ-Health* **48**(5): 328–335.

Hoek G. and Brunekreef B. (1994) Effects of low-level winter air pollution concentrations on respiratory health of Dutch children. *Environ-Res* **64**(2): 136–150.

Hoek G., Brunekreef B., Goldbohm S., Fischer P. and Brandt P.A. van den. (2002) Association between mortality and indicators of traffic-related air pollution in the Netherlands: A cohort study. *Lancet* **360**: 1203–1209.

Hoek G., Verhoeff A.P. and Fisher P.H. (1997) Daily mortality and air pollution in the Netherlands, 1986–1994. Wageningen: Report Agricultural University Wageningen.

Hoffman F.O. and Hammonds J.S. (1994) Propagation of uncertainty in risk assessments: The need to distinguish between uncertainty due to lack of knowledge and uncertainty due to variability. *Risk Anal* **14**: 707–712.

Hofstetter P. and Hammitt J.K. (2002) Selecting human health metrics for environmental decision-support tools. *Risk Analy* **22**: 965–983.

Hollander A.E.M. de. (2003) Are the costs and benefits in balance? In van Oers (eds). Health on course. Public health status and forecasts report 2002. Bohn Stafleu Van Loghum, Houten.

Holland M., Berry J. and Foster D. (eds). Externalities of Energy. Volume 7: Methodology 1998 update. Brussels: European Commission, Directorate-General XII, Science, Research and Development, 1998.

Hollander A.E.M. de, Melse J.M., Lebret E. and Kramers P.G.N. (1999) An aggregate public health indicator to represent the impact of multiple environmental exposures. *Epidemiol* **10**: 606–617.

Hollander A.E.M., Preller E.A., Heisterkamp S., Dusseldorp A., Amelink C.B. and Brunekreef B. Hospital admission and ER visits due to ozone air pollution: An empirical Bayesian approach to quantitative review. Bilthoven: RIVM Annual report, 1998.

Hollander A.E.M. de and Staatsen B.A.M. (2003) Health, environment and quality of life: An epidemiological perspective on urban development. *Landscape, Urban Planning* **989**: 1–10.

Hurley J. (2000) An overview of the normative economics of the health sector. In Culyer A.J., Newhouse JP (eds). *Handbook of Health Economics.* Vol. 1. Elsevier, Amsterdam, 56–118.

Institute for Environmental Studies. Economic evaluation of air quality targets for sulphur dioxide, nitrogen dioxide, fine and suspended particulates and lead. Final report European Commision, DG XI, Amsterdam: IVM, 1997.

Janssen N.A.H., Hoek G., Brunekreef B., Harssema H., Mensink I. and Zuidhof A. (1998) Personal sampling of PM_{10} among adults: Relations between personal, indoor and outdoor concentrations. *Am J Epidemiol* **147**: 537–547.

Jones-Lee M. (1985) The value of safety: Results from a national sample survey. *Econom J* **95**: 49–72.

Klose T. (1999) The contingent valuation method in health care. *Health Policy* **47**: 97–123.

Krahn M.D., Berka C., Langlois P. and Detsky A.S. (1996) Direct and indirect costs of asthma in Canada, 1990. *Can Med Assoc J* **154**: 821–831.

Krewski D., Burnett R.T., Goldberg M.S., *et al.* Reanalysis of the Hravard Six Cities Study and the American Cancer Society Study of particulate air pollution and mortality, special report. Cambridge, MA: Health Effects Institute, 2000.

Krupnick A.J. and Portney P.R. (1991) Controlling urban air pollution: A benefit-cost assessment. *Science* **252**: 522–528.

Kruppnick A.J. and Cropper M.L. (1992) The effect of information on health risk valuations. *J Risk Uncertainty* **5**: 29–48.

Künzli N., Kaiser R., Medina S., Studnicka M., Filiger P., Herry M., Horak F. Jr., Puybonnieux-Texier V., Quénel P., Schneider J., Seethaler R., Vergnaud J.-C. and Sommer H. (2000) Public health impact of outdoor and traffic related air pollution: A European assessment. *Lancet* **356**: 795–801.

Künzli N., Medina S., Kaiser R., Quenel P., Horak F. Jr. and Studnicka M. (2001) Assessment of deaths attributable to air pollution: Should we use risk estimates based on time series or on cohort studies? *Am J Epidemiol* **153**(11): 1050–1055.

Laboratory for Air Pollution Research, RIVM. Air Quality. Annual Report 2002 (in Dutch). Bilthoven: RIVM, report n.o. 725301009, 2003.

Leksell I. and Rabl A. (2001) Air pollution and mortality: Quantification and valuation of years of life lost. *Risk Anal* **21**: 843–857.

Lipfert F.W., Perry H.M. Jr., Miller J.P., Baty J.D., Wyzga R.E. and Carmody S.E. (2003) Air pollution, blood pressure, and their long-term associations with mortality. *Inhal-Toxicol* **15**(5): 493–512.

Melse J.M. and Hollander A.E.M de. Environment and health within the OECD region: Lost health, lost money. Background document to the OECD Environmental Outlook. Bilthoven: RIVM, report 402101 001, 2001.

Melse J.M. and Kramers P.G.N. Calculation of disease burden in the Netherlands (in Dutch). Bilthoven: RIVM, report 4315001028, 1998 (English version submitted for publication, 1999).

Ministry of Health. Mortality and morbidity during the London fog o.f., December 1952. Reports on Public Health and Medical Subjects N.o. 95. HMSO: London. 1954.

Ministry of Housing, Physical Planning and Environmental Protection. Premises for Risk Management (annex to the Netherlands National Environmental Policy Plan 1990–1994). The Hague: Ministry of VROM, 1989.

Morgan M.G. (1993) Risk analysis and management. *Sci Am* July: 24–30.

Morgan M.G. (2000) Risk management should be about efficiency and equity. *Environ Sci Technol* **34** (1): 32A–34A.

Murray C.J.L. and Lopez A.D. (eds). The global burden of disease; A comprehensive assessment of mortality and disability from disease, injury, and risk factors in 1990 and projected to 2020. Global burden of disease and injury series, Vol. I. Harvard University Press, 1996.

Murray C.J.L. and Rethinking D.A.L.Y.s. In Murray C.J.L. and Lopez A.D. (eds). The global burden of disease; a comprehensive assessment of mortality and disability from disease, injury, and risk factors in 1990 and projected to 2020. Global burden of disease and injury series, Vol. I. Harvard University Press, 1996.

National Instittute of Public Health and the Environment (RIVM). 5th National Environmental Outlook, 2000–2030. Alphen a/d Rijn: Samson b.v., 2000.

National Institute of Public Health and the Environment. National Environmental Outlook 2000–2030. Alphen a/d Rijn: Samnson b.v., 2000.

National Research Council. Risk Assessment in the Federal Government: Managing the Process. National Academy Press, Washington DC: 1983.

Navrud S. Valuing health impacts from air pollution in Europe: New empirical evidence on Morbidity. Norway: Agricultural University of Norway; Working Paper, 1997.

Nevalainen J. and Pekkanen J. (1998) The effect of particulate air pollution on life expectancy. *Sci Total Environ* **217**: 137–141.

Nord E. Cost-value analysis in health care: Making sense out of QALYs. Cambridge, UK: Cambridge University Press, 1999.

Olsen J.A. and Smith R.D. (2001) Theory versus practice: A review of 'willingness-to-pay' in health and health care, *Health Econ* **10**(1): 39–52.

Ostro B. and Chestnut L. (1998) Assessing the Health benefits of reducing particulate matter air pollution in the United States. *Environ Res* **76**: 94–106.

Pope C.A. 3rd, Burnett R.T., Thun M.J., Calle E.E., Krewski D., Ito K. and Thurston G.D. (2002) Lung cancer, cardiopulmonary mortality, and long-term exposure to fine particulate air pollution. *JAMA* **287**(9): 1132–1141.

Pope III C.A., Thun M.J., Namboodiri M.M., Dockery D.W., Evans J.S., Speizer F.E. and Health C.W. (1995) Particulate air pollution as a predictor of mortality in a prospective study of US adults. *Am J Respir Crit Care Med* **151**: 669–674.

Pope III C.A., Thun M.J., Namboodiri M.M., Dockery D.W., Evans J.S., Speizer F.E. and Health C.W. (1995) Particulate air pollution as a predictor of mortality in a prospective study of US adults. *Am J Respir Crit Care Med* **151**: 669–674.

Roemer W., Hoek G. and Brunekreef B. (1993) Effect of ambient winter air pollution on respiratory health of children with chronic respiratory symptoms. *Am Rev Respir Dis* **147**(1): 118–124.

Roemer W., Hoek G. and Brunekreef B. (2000) Pollution effects on asthmatic individuals in Europe: The PEACE-study. *Clin Exp Allergy* **30**: 1067–75.

Ruwaard D. and Kramers P.G.N. (eds). Public Health Status and Forecasts 1997. Health, prevention and health care in the Netherlands until 2015. Bilthoven/Maarssen, the Netherlands: National Institute of Public Health and the Environment, Elsevier/de Tijdstroom, 1998.

Ruwaard D., Kramers P.G.N. Public Health Status and Forecasts (2) "Som der delen" (in Dutch, English version in prep). Maarssen: National Institute of Public Health and the Environment, Elsevier/de Tijdstroom, 1997.

Saltman R.B., Figueras J. (eds). European health Care Reform: Analysis of current strategies. World Health Organisation; Copenhagen: Regional publications, European series; no 72, 1997.

Schayck C.P. van Dompeling E., Herwaarden C.L.A. van Folgering H., Hoogen H.J.M. and van den Weel C. van. Degree of bronchial hyper-responsiveness, an indicator of the severity of chronic bronchitis and asthma. In CP van Schayk. Dissertation, Nijmegen University, 199?

Schwartz J. (1993) Particulate air pollution and chronic respiratory disease. *Environ Res* **62**: 7–13.

Schwartz J. (1994) What are people dying of on high air pollution days. *Environ Res* **64**: 26–35.

Schwartz J. (1998, 2000) Harvesting and long term exposure effects in the relation between air pollution and mortality. *Am J Epidemiol* **151**: 440–448. *et al. Am J Resp Crit Car Med* **157**: A879.

Slovic P. (1999) Trust, emtion, sex, politics, and science: Surveying the risk-assessment battlefield. *Risk-Anal.* **19**(4): 689–701.

Stouthard M.E.A., Essink-Bot M.L., Bonsel G.J., Barendregt J.J., Kramers P.G.N., Water H.P.A. van de, Gunning-Schepers and Maas PJ van der. Disability weights for diseases in the Netherlands. Rotterdam: Dept. of Public Health, Erasmus University, 1997.

Taylor W.R. and Newacheck P.W. (1992) Impact of childhood asthma on health. *Pediatrics* **90**: 657–662.

Ten Berge W.F. and Stallen P.J.M. (1995) How to compare risk assessments for accidental and chronic exposure. *Risk Anal* **15**: 111–113.

Tengs T.O., Adams M.E., Pliskin J.S., Gelb Safran D., Siegel J.E., Weinstein M.C. and Graham J.D. (1995) Five-hundred life-saving interventions and their cost-effectiveness. *Risk Anal* **15**: 369–390.

Thompson K.M., Burmaster D.E. and Crouch E.A. (1992) Monte Carlo techniques for quantitative uncertainty analysis in public health risk assessments. *Risk Anal* **12**: 53–63.

Towse A., Pritchard C. and Devlin N. Cost-effectiveness Thresholds. Economic and ethical issues. King's Fund and Office of Health Economics, London: 2002.

USEPA. Air quality guidelines for particulate matter. Washington DC: US Environmental Protection Agency, 1996.

U.S. Environmental Protection Agency. Regulatory impact analysis for proposed particulate matter national ambient air quality standards. Research Triangle Park, NC, 1996.

US Environmental Protection Agency: Innovative strategies and economics group, Office of Air Quality Planning and Standards. Regulatory Impact Analysis for proposed particulate matter national ambient air quality standard. Research Triangle Park: US EPA, 1996.

Vedal S. (1997) Ambient particles and health: Lines that divide. *J Air Waste Manag Assoc* **47**: 551–581.

Viscusi W.K., Magat W.A. and Huber J. (1991) Pricing environmental health risks: Survey assessment of risk-risk and risk-dollar trade-offs for chronic bronchitis. *J Environ Econom Manag* **21**: 32–51.

Wit G.A. de, Busschbach J.J.V. and de Charro F.T.H. (2000) Sensitivity and perspective in the valuation of health status: Who's values count? *Health Econom* **9**: 109–126.

World Bank. World Development Report 1993: Investing in Health — World Development Indicators. Oxford University Press, New York: 1993.

World Bank. World Development Report 1993: Investing in Health — World Development Indicators. Oxford University Press, New York: 1993.

World Health Organization. Air quality guidelines for Europe. Copenhagen: WHO Regional Office for Europe; Regional Publications, European Series no 23, 1987.

World Health Organization. Air quality guidelines for Europe. WHO, Copenhagen: 2nd edn. European series, No 95, 2000.

World Health Organisation: WHO Working group. Health aspects of air pollution with particulate matter, ozone and nitrogen dioxide. WHO: Bonn, 2003.

Zanobetti A., Schwartz J., Samoli E., *et al.* (2002) The temporal pattern of mortality responses to air pollution: A multi-city assessment of mortality displacement. *Epidemiol* **13**: 87–93.

Zeger S.L., Dominici F. and Samet J. (1999) Harvesting-resistant estimates of air pollution effects of mortality. *Epidemiol* **10**: 171–175.

INDEX